Terror on the Screen

Also by New Academia Publishing

Terror on the Screen

Witnesses and the Re-animation of 9/11
as Image-event,
Popular Culture,
and Pornography

Luke Howie

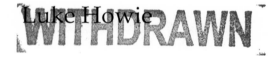

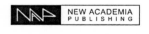
NEW ACADEMIA
PUBLISHING

Washington, DC

Library of Congress Control Number: 2010934626
ISBN 978-0-9828061-3-5 paperback (alk. paper)

New Academia Publishing
PO Box 27420, Washington, DC
info@newacademia.com - www.newacademia.com

Contents

Illustrations   vi

Preface   vii

Acknowledgements   ix

Part I: Witnesses and the Re-animation of 9/11 as an Image-event   1

   1. Witnessing Terrorism   3

   2. Welcome to the City, Welcome to the Desert of the Real   33

   3. Celebrity Terrorism: Passion for the Real   61

Part II: 9/11 as Popular Culture and Pornography   87

   4. Representing Terrorism: Re-animating Post-9/11 New York City   89

   5. They Were Created By Man ... and They Have a Plan: Subjective and Objective Violence in *Battlestar Galactica* and the War on Terror   111

   6. Post-9/11 Comedy/Trauma   135

   7. Terrorsex: Witnesses, Spectacular Terrorism and Pornography   175

   8. A Screen Culture of Terrorism   203

Notes   225

Bibliography   258

Index   277

Illustrations

Twin Towers, by Brendan Rose, courtesy of Brian Rose,   vii
New York City. Used with permission.

View of Melbourne   30

Etihad Stadium   44

Rialto   44

Southern Cross Station   45

The Age Building   45

Preface

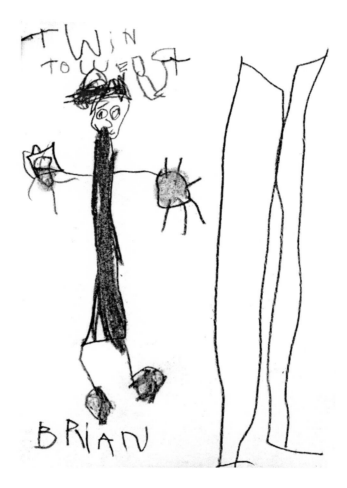

This image was drawn by a New Yorker. But the artist was too young to remember 11 September 2001. He did not witness it in real-time (as far as he knows), but he is growing up as a New Yorker in the post-9/11 world as a first generation survivor in a city targeted by international terrorism. The image appears on his father's online journal. It was here that I encountered these witnesses of 9/11.

As Piaget and others have shown, young children have a keen sense of images and imagery. It is a sense that gradually becomes socialized into symbolic norms and frames. As children draw they are engaged with complex semiotic networks that can offer extraordinary insight into everyday, even unconscious, realities. This particular image is both simple yet powerful, not only for what it depicts, but because it was drawn by a seven year-old five years after 9/11. He did not need to witness 9/11 to understand its meanings and consequences – it was part of his city, part of his world and part of his identity whether he wanted it to be or not. He is, after all, a New Yorker. His father, a photographer, is in the image holding a camera. Even at such a young age, the relationship between the camera's lens and 9/11 is obvious to him. He is a witness unlike any other I have encountered.

Yet, this artist and I are not so unalike. We were both witnesses, we have both watched, even though he lives in New York City and I live in Melbourne, Australia. Whilst I cannot understand what 9/11 means to this young artist his drawing gives me a clue. It is an insight. Perhaps most incredible about this image is that the Twin Towers are still standing – the opposite of his experience of being a post-9/11 New Yorker. The Towers may have been airbrushed out of some post-9/11 television in an act of disavowal, but this child perhaps has little need for forgetfulness. He has faced it. He has a story to tell. He is the witness.

Acknowledgements

Terror on the Screen is a culmination of complex histories and realities of watching films, television, reading books, mining the internet, witnessing terrorism, the news media, the entertainment habits of cosmopolitan citizens of major cities, the production decisions of television creators and directors, the actors that play the roles and inhabit the stories, and those who watch. This book is also about violence, terror, death and destruction, and how these things are represented on the screen and in our imagination. As such, I cannot name everyone who has made this book possible. But there are those who were close by as I wrote this book. Some participated in production by reading drafts and offering advice and comments. Others encouraged me as I researched and wrote. One was my inspiration.

I would like to thank my colleagues in Behavioural Studies and the School of Political and Social Inquiry at Monash University. Peter Kelly, Nicky Pitt and Perri Campbell offered thoughtful comments during the book's development and read several drafts. They challenged me to think about this project in new and complex ways. Peter Kelly is my mentor. Without his daily advice, motivation and coaching this book, indeed any of my work, would certainly not exist. Thanks to Francesca Collins, Roseanne Misajon, Greg Barton, Pete Lentini, Gary Bouma, Irfan Ahmad, Ben MacQueen, Denise Cuthbert, Nel Halloran, Colleen Lewis, Dennis Woodward, Waleed Aly, all of the crew from the Global Terrorism Research Centre

(GTReC), Paul A. Taylor, Gavin Kendall, Keith Abbott, Athol Yates, Stuart Koschade, Chad Whelan and a host of graduate students for your support. These people have all made important contributions to my career and this book through their support and encouragement.

To friends and family – the people who are my companions in witnessing screen cultures. Perri Campbell, Maree Luckman, Maddison Howie, Elle Howie, Margaret Campbell, Craig Campbell, Chantelle Campbell, Hamish Campbell, Margaret Luckman, John Luckman, Lindsay Wise, Kaine Leonard, Chris Henderson, Lawrence and Kathryn Obaldo, Shannon Hyder and Nick Hyder. Thanks for reminding me of movies, actors, quotes, events, non-events and websites. These people together are both my life and a powerful pop-culture encyclopedia.

Chapter four of this book first appeared in volume three, number three of the *International Journal of Žižek Studies* as "Representing Terrorism: Reanimating Post-9/11 New York City" (http://zizekstudies.org/). It is used here with permission. This chapter was also delivered as a paper to The Australian Sociological Association (TASA) conference in Melbourne in 2008. Thanks to the audience for their aggressive questions and comments.

An earlier version of chapter five also first appeared in volume five, number one of the *International Journal of Žižek Studies*. Many thanks go to Paul A. Taylor and an anonymous reviewer for their excellent advice that improved this chapter significantly.

This book is dedicated to my inspiration, Perri Campbell. Life companion, number one fan and the most talented scholar I have ever met.

Part I

Witnesses and the Re-animation of 9/11 as an Image-event

1.

Witnessing Terrorism

MULDER: What's wrong?

SCULLY: Well, I just climbed up twelve floors, I'm hot, I'm thirsty and to be honest, I'm wondering what I'm doing up here.

MULDER: You're looking for a bomb.

SCULLY: Yes, I know that, but the threat was called in to the federal building across the street.

MULDER: I think they have that covered.

SCULLY: Mulder, when a terrorist bomb threat is called in, the rational purpose of providing that information is to allow us to find the bomb. The rational object of terrorism is to promote terror. If you'd study the statistics, you'd find the model behavioral pattern for virtually every case where a threat has turned up an explosive device; and if we don't act in accordance with that data, if you ignore it as we have done, the chances are great that if there actually is a bomb, we might not find it. Lives could be lost ...

MULDER: Whatever happened to playing a hunch, Scully? The element of surprise? Random acts of unpredictability? If we fail to anticipate the unforeseen or expect the unexpected in a universe of infinite possibilities, we may find ourselves at the mercy of anyone or anything that cannot be programmed, categorized or easily referenced.[1]

This book is about how terrorism is witnessed, spectacularized, interpreted and remembered. It is about what happens after horrific and spectacular images of terrorism are captured by the global news media and distributed to audiences of witnesses. In this book, I want to map a path that begins with violent acts of terrorism and ends with *terror on the screen*. This pathway is littered with witnesses both near and far from terrorism's "flashpoint",[2] popular, tele-visual and screen cultures involving political satire and counter-cultures, traumascapes, a terror-voyeurism that is akin to watching pornography, the news media and its news junkies, and furious bloggers spewing vitriol and racism. On this pathway I found many things. Saviors of humanity named Morpheus and Neo. Terror celebrities and celebrity cultures. Six friends having coffee in Manhattan. Post-9/11 cartoons that encourage us to laugh at the post-9/11 world. Cylons. A posse of sexy secret agents. A porn-star named Jenna Jamison and a place called "Imaginationland" where our imaginations were targeted by terrorists, and subsequently ran wild. These are all important artifacts of a post-9/11 screen culture.

This book is also, in many respects, about the 11 September 2001 terrorist attacks in New York City, Washington DC and a field in Shanksville, Pennsylvania. It is about some of the extraordinary consequences of these attacks. "9/11" entered the world as an image – a spectacle – for many millions of people throughout the world. Many millions witnessed the attacks in real-time, live on television. As the consequences of 9/11 have endured in international wars fought in its name, in acts of brutality and torture, in further acts of terrorism, in politics and elections, so too have the spectacular images of 9/11. These images have been replayed incessantly, routinely reanimated on television and computer screens, and 9/11 has quickly become one of the most witnessed events in tele-visual history. These images, and their consequences, have endured.

This endurance has coincided with considerable efforts to understand, research, explore, evaluate, quantify, qualify and gain knowledge about 9/11. This book is one such effort, but it is not one that is routinely attempted. It is far more likely that those who write books about terrorism will focus on the who, why, how and when of terrorism than on how terrorism is *witnessed, spectacular-ized, interpreted and remembered*. It is perhaps even less likely that the subject of a book about terrorism would be popular, tele-visual and screen cultures. As Special Agents Fox Mulder and Dana Scully stand atop the wrong building, searching for a terrorist bomb that is not supposed to be there, they gain a different perspective, they work against the prescribed method and course of action, they invert many of the assumptions that have been made about terrorism and terrorists. Standing on the wrong building, "playing a hunch", can have its advantages.

Like Mulder, I followed a "hunch". I became aware of a 9/11 that I had not immediately seen, that I did not witness (at first), that I had trouble categorizing. I witnessed 9/11 live on television. I witnessed the news coverage in the days that followed. The images were spectacular and horrific – I felt an uncomfortable combination of disgust, a type of grotesque excitement and an overwhelming discomfort at the sight of the death and destruction. The whole event was drowned out with images. Soon after, I witnessed comedy talk shows return to the air. I witnessed David Letterman's and John Stewart's emotional accounts of 9/11. I witnessed popular television shows, some set in New York City, return to the air. But these television programs betrayed any hope of a quick return to normal. When *Friends* returned for the eighth season in late September 2001 something was missing. It took me a few moments to process the reality that the Twin Towers, which had once littered the background images of the opening credits and the scene transitions, were gone. Other situation comedies set in New York City followed suit. What interested me most was that despite the removal of the Twin Towers, life in these television programs, the lives of the fictional characters living in NYC, continued uninterrupted. It was as though 9/11 had never happened. Simply and quietly the Twin Towers were airbrushed out of the shot, as though their disappearance had not been dramatic and globally witnessed, as though the Towers slipped away in the night. Other programs tackled 9/11 head-on. The *West Wing* featured a post-9/11 storyline. *Battlestar Galactica* was re-imagined in a post-9/11 world. And it was not long before feature films about 9/11 were commonplace in the world's cinemas. Indeed, it was not long until *The Simpsons, Family Guy* and *South Park* even had us laughing at the post-9/11 world.

Some might say that this is not the best way to understand the meanings and consequences of 9/11. Perhaps I am standing on the wrong building. But I do so in the hope of finding something new, something different, something that has been dismissed as less interesting or less important. I want to show that the ways that terrorism is witnessed, spectacularized, interpreted and remembered is important. I want to show that popular, tele-visual and screen cultures are important artifacts of the post-9/11 world. In standing on the wrong building I am not alone, nor am I the first. In fact, I am in good company. The prominent terrorism studies academic Walter Laqueur observed in 1987 that "Fiction holds some promise for the understanding of the terrorist phenomenon".[3] In arguing his case for taking fiction and popular culture seriously, he warned of the rigidity of "the study of terrorism as practiced by political scientists" but called for care in moving from a study of terrorism as a "science" towards the study of terrorism through the "arts".[4] Such a move, in Laqueur's view, represents a transition from the realm of "relative certainties" to the "realm of impression".[5] These "impressions" are undoubtedly important. As John Tulloch – a media academic and a victim of the London "7/7" bombings – argued, media representations of terrorism play a vital social and cultural role after a terrorist attack. He writes of screen cultures after 7/7; "whatever public channel of communication they adopt, they are all important, vocal parts of a groundswell of alternative political voices … They all engage directly with … an international culture of fear … [and] are asking questions about an alternative democracy of ethical responsibility and civic engagement".[6]

For Laqueur the movement from relative certainty to the realm of impression promises to make some absences in the study of terrorism presences, whilst making current presences absent. Whilst my book will offer little to improve knowledge of how terrorist attacks can be prevented, how terrorists become radicalized and how they might be rehabilitated, it will illuminate other fields where terrorism studies knowledge is lacking. Examining popular, tele-visual and screen cultures of terrorism in the post-9/11 world can tell us much about how terrorism is represented, produced and re-produced and how terrorism is *witnessed* throughout the world. By making traditional fields of counterterrorism and terrorism research less visible, I bring the experience of terrorism's witnesses to the foreground.

I seek to highlight witnessing by making popular, tele-visual and screen cultures of terrorism more visible. In doing so I want to signal some important signposts of post-9/11 screen culture. These signposts are necessarily contextual and situated, and dependent upon the vantage point of every witness. But 9/11's witnesses also have much in common. My goal is to find "new and adequate ways of thinking *of*, *about* and *for* the world we live in"[7], a world that can indefinitely be described as *post-9/11*. But before I outline how I will tackle the post-9/11 screen cultural artifacts I have chosen for analysis in this book, I want to show how the role of the witness has always been an underlying concern for understanding our world and for understanding terrorism. The witness is central to any understanding of terrorism, although this is seldom acknowledged. But, as I will show in the next section, the witness has played a central role in the history of terrorism and in attempts to settle on a terrorism definition. The witness, in this way, is the first and most important absence I want to highlight and draw into presence.

The Witness

The witness is the central figure of this book. I base my arguments in this book on the assumption that to witness terrorism is to be a victim of terrorism since, as Jenkins has argued, terrorists want a lot of people watching, not just a lot of people dead.[8] Those who watch, those who bear witness, are the intended targets of terrorism. Those who die in terrorist attacks are means to an end in the terrorists' desire for attention and celebrity. For Haraway[9] the witness holds a paradoxically powerful and vulnerable place in the social and cultural world. The foundation of witnessing for Haraway is being a part of a "collective", "networked" and "situated" visual practice:

> Witnessing is seeing; attesting; standing publicly accountable for, and psychically vulnerable to, one's visions and representations. Witnessing is a collective, limited practice that depends on the constructed and never finished credibility of those who do it, all of whom are mortal, fallible, and fraught with the consequences of unconscious and disowned desires and fears. [10]

As a witness and researcher of 9/11, I inhabit the many stories of 9/11 that I encounter in the post-9/11 world. I inhabit the story of participating in a reading group on the seventh anniversary of 9/11 and the momentarily threatening passenger airplane flying near Melbourne's skyline. I inhabit George W. Bush's address to the American people on the same anniversary. I inhabit the television programs that feature images and imagery of 9/11, terrorism, security and fear. And I am not the only one.

The witnessing that I explore in this book has been formed through partial connections, complex relationships and problematic fusions between witnesses and audiences and popular, tele-visual and screen cultures. Donna Haraway has described situations where such multiple connections form with the metaphor of the "cat's cradle" game in which participants make "string figures" on fingers.[11]

> Cat's cradle is about patterns and knots; the game takes great skill and can result in some serious surprises. One person can build up a large repertoire of string figures on a single pair of hands, but the cat's cradle figures can be passed back and forth on hands of several players, who add new moves in the building of complex patterns. Cat's cradle invites a sense of collective work, of one person not being able to make all the patterns alone … It is not always possible to repeat interesting patterns, and figuring out what happened to result in intriguing patterns is an embodied analytical skill. [12]

I intend to play a type of cat's cradle game in this book in order to uncover patterns of 9/11, terrorism, security and fear in post-9/11 screen cultures. Joining me in this endeavor are a variety of figures in the post-9/11 world that include human respondents in social research in Melbourne, Australia; respondents to newspaper articles and terror-events in the blogosphere; television shows, films and those who have written about them; the characters in these shows and films; fashion photographers; techniques of social research and the associated methods; literary traditions of critical social theory; and the people I encounter and speak to about 9/11 and terrorism when I am at work, at home, in the city, and traveling the world.

Valid witnessing depends not only on modesty but also on nurturing and acknowledging alliances with a lively array of others, who are like and unlike, human and not, inside and outside what have been the defended boundaries of hegemonic selves and powerful places.[13]

Witnessing is a crucial force for understanding the meanings and consequences of terrorism. Witnessing is embodied, situated and located and it is through witnesses that we discover that "Understanding the world is about living inside stories".[14]

Witnessing is, however, a deeply problematic phenomenon. It is a differing, subjective and dependent experience. The unreliability of our visual skills has the potential to make a study of witnessing a study of conjecture. Vision is an "embodied" practice that makes witnessing possible.[15] But our over reliance on our problematic visual capacity – a visual capacity that, according to cognitive and neuro-scientific explanations, functions through the eyes first capturing stimuli that is then interpreted by the brain where some things are emphasized and other things are ignored – means that we have trusted our vision to "leap out of the marked body and into a conquering gaze from nowhere".[16] As Haraway so powerfully puts it:

The eyes have been used to signify a perverse capacity – honed to perfection in the history of science tied to militarism, capitalism, colonialism, and male supremacy – to distance the knowing subject from everybody and everything in the interests of unfettered power. The instruments of visualization in multinationalist, postmodern culture have compounded these meanings of dis-embodiment. The visualizing technologies are without apparent limit; the eye of any ordinary primate like us can be endlessly enhanced by sonography systems, magnetic resonance imaging, artificial intelligence-linked graphic manipulation systems, scanning electron microscopes, computer-aided tomography scanners, colour enhancement techniques, satellite surveillance systems, home and office VDTs, a camera for every purpose.[17]

This visual "technological feast" has armed the witness with the tools to indulge in visually "unregulated gluttony" where "all perspective gives way to infinitely mobile vision, which no longer seems just mythically about the god-trick of seeing everything from nowhere, but to have put the myth into ordinary practice".[18]   On and after 9/11 this has translated to a capacity to witness, capture, record, and replay over and over again 9/11, other acts of terror and their consequences. Witnessing 9/11 and other acts of contemporary terror are little more than a Google away. Moreover, this visual capturing and replaying – or *re-animating* – has made post-9/11 screen culture possible. John Urry has seemingly picked up on this theme in relating visualized screen culture and the 9/11 terrorist attacks:

> The whole world watched the surreal moment as planes with live passengers flew into and demolished two of the largest buildings in the world. The World Trade Center, a city in the air, was with two strokes bombed out of existence, an "uncanny" moment when the distinction between fantasy and reality was effaced in astonishing images, eclipsing anything Hollywood has generated.[19]

What these forces – witnessing, the dominance of the visual sense, and the ability to capture and record imagery – amount to are the coordinates of a victimized audience in the theater of terrorism. This is who we are; imperfect human actors with unreliable visual capacities that do more to foster conjecture than accurate or unified perceptions. Perhaps our best hope is to understand as many stories as possible. Indeed, these imperfect human actors are the true targets of terrorism. They are the receivers and responders to the terrorist's violent message. The witness of terrorism has always played a central role in understanding the meanings and consequences of terrorism, even if that role has tended to lay hidden in terrorism scholarship and analysis. It is to this scholarship that I now turn.

Witnesses in the Theater of Terrorism

Many writers and scholars in the "terrorism studies" canon have argued that terrorism has changed significantly throughout history in terms of methods and tactics, the targets and the victims chosen, the ideology that drives the attacks, and the way that the word "terrorism" has been used.[20] What it means to be a witness and a victim of terrorism has also changed significantly, but some consistency nonetheless remains – the more spectacular the act of terrorism, the greater the audience of witnesses in the theater of terrorism. Walter Laqueur once argued that terrorism "has been a tragedy for the victims, but seen in an historical perspective it seldom has been more than a nuisance".[21] But the terrorism of 9/11 and many other post-9/11 attacks call this claim into question. What Laqueur's argument fails to adequately account for is the role of the image in generating spectacular terrorism that is witnessed large distances from terrorism's *flashpoint*.

Indeed, a close inspection of the literature exploring the history of terrorism shows that terrorists have always held the "witness" as the highest priority. What it also reveals is that goals such as political change, ideological upheaval or religious influence have often been secondary goals to the ultimate desire to have people watch the violence. Yet, when witnesses watch, these secondary goals are advanced by the spectacular terrorism image-event. Because of this, I suggest that the term "victim" is often misunderstood in the terrorism studies literature. Often, exploring the meaning of the "victims" of terrorism amounts to an uncritical reference to those who perish or who are injured in an act of terrorism and their families. But these "victims" of terrorism are instruments to achieving the greater goal of publicity and reaching audiences of witnesses. Terrorism has always been theater for the living. Terror groups such as the *Sicarii*, the *Hashashin* and the *Thuggee* – groups that did not have the ability to generate spectacular tele-visual events – were able to create violent *imagery* in the minds of witnesses. Stories about their violent attacks quickly spread and instilled terror in anyone who heard the tales both near to and far from where their attacks occurred.[22] The Sicarii were an extreme Jewish faction that became active in the first century CE during the Roman occupation of Palestine. Their tactic was to attack in the crowds that gathered during holidays and religious festivals. Their targets were mostly moneylenders, priests and other Jews that they believed were collaborating with the occupying Romans.[23] Their ostensible goal was to overthrow Roman rule and establish self-governance. Their method for achieving this was to spread terror and fear amongst witnesses. Their attention seeking terror was often combined with organized guerrilla attacks launched against strategic Roman positions from Sicarii camps and strongholds in the countryside. The crowds in which the killings took place became frenzied as news of Sicarii attacks spread. The Sicarii desired publicity for their cause and were successful in inspiring an uprising. The historian Josephus wrote that the "Sicarii committed murders in broad daylight in the heart of Jerusalem".[24] News of their exploits often travelled to distant audiences.

The Hashashin were a radical Muslim sect that targeted rulers and religious leaders that they believed were corrupt. The Hashashin were responsible for the deaths of many prominent religious figures and leaders.[25] In 1090, the Hashashin seized the fortress of Alamut and, several years later, completed assassinations of the Sultan of Baghdad, Nazim al Mulq, Count Raymond II of Tripoli and Marquis Conrad of Montferrat, ruler of Jerusalem.[26] They became well known in many regions for carrying out bold and brazen attacks against high profile targets and for their supposed love of the drug hashish. It was popularly believed that the assassins would get high on the drug before embarking on a mission, although accounts on this differ. The Hashashin carried out assassinations to achieve their various political goals, but they were also concerned with attracting witnesses and gaining publicity. Rapoport has argued that they did not need mass communication and media to reach witnesses in distant locations.[27] Their prominent "victims" were murdered "in venerated sites and royal courts" on holy days and during festivals to guarantee that there would be many witnesses and that word of their actions and purpose would spread. In this way, they posed a physical threat to those who were their targets and an emotional and psychological threat to all who heard the tales and accepted the imagery created by the stories that were told of their violence. Some Hashashin terrorists, after carrying out an assassination, would remain and accept their inevitable fate as guards and soldiers struck them down. This defied reason for witnesses to their violence and for those who heard the tales.[28] Stories of the Hashashin's violence reached fantastic heights. As these stories and their notoriety spread they became deeply feared.

The Thuggee first became active in the seventh century and were particularly well-known for their violent attacks during the thirteenth century in what is present-day India.[29] The Thuggee were not attempting to influence any group. Rather, they were committing murders they believed satisfied their deity: the Hindu goddess Kali.[30] The Thugs were not directly motivated by a desire to attract witnesses or gain publicity. Their terror was not carried out to achieve a greater goal and audiences of witnesses. Their violence was an end in itself. They nonetheless generated powerful terror and audiences of witnesses who heard of tales of the Thuggee. News of their attacks spread far and wide and, like the Hashashin, their violence, which involved ritual desecrations of their "victims", was perceived to be appalling and irrational. The spectacle of Thuggee terrorism generated enduring folklore and legend.[31] The terrorisms of these groups were indeed powerful. The fact that they are still discussed in journals and books is testament to their influence.

Whilst only the eye-witnesses to attacks carried out by these groups *literally* viewed the violence, the stories of Sicarii, Hashashin and Thuggee terror spread their message to a wider audience with terrifying and powerful imagery. In the 21st century the message and the desire to gain attention remains relatively unchanged but the method of dissemination has changed significantly. Internet and satellite communication technologies allowed the 9/11 terrorist attacks to gain an audience not just through storytelling but as a spectacular, globalized image-event. But 9/11 and these historical moments of terror share the capacity of terrorism to attract an audience, a watcher, a witness. However, in much of the literature examining terrorism the techniques, tactics, the perpetrators and their motivations are – understandably – the emphasis. Far too little scholarly endeavor has focused on the role of witnesses who are the targets of terrorism. The comparative silence in examining the role of the witness in understanding terrorism is especially evident in literature that defines terrorism.

Rapoport has argued that "virtually all modern conceptions of terrorism assume that the perpetrators only mean to harm their victims incidentally. The principal object is the public, whose consciousness will be aroused by the outrage".[32] Yet a study by Weinberg et al. that examines 73 definitions of terrorism up until 2002, all of which were developed before 9/11, to assess the elements that were most frequently included shows that the witness is only occasionally considered part of the definitional picture.[33] The authors compared their findings with a similar study from Schmid and Jongman in 1988.[34] Of the 22 elements in terrorism definitions identified by Weinberg et al., the role of the witness is prominent in only five. These five elements are: a fear and terror outcome; psychological effects and reactions; victim/victimized distinctions (where the victims are killed or injured in the attack, and the victimized are the witnesses); publicity; and symbolism. Interestingly the role of the witness in terrorism definitions decreased significantly from 1988 to 2002. Where the 1988 survey reported "fear and terror" appearing in 51% of definitions, in the 2002 study it appeared in only 22%. In 1988, "psychological effects" appeared in 41.5% of definitions – in 2002 it appeared in only 5.5%. The "victim/victimized" distinction was featured in 37.5% of definitions in the 1988 study, but in only 25% in the 2002 study. "Publicity" was a feature in 21.5% of definitions in the 1988 study, and 18% in the 2002 study. Finally, "symbolism" was a feature of 13.5% of definitions in the 1988 study, and only in 5.5% in the 2002 study. The analysis of Weinberg et al. can therefore be used to suggest that the role of the witness in defining terrorism has diminished since 1988. Post-9/11 definitions, however, were not considered in Weinberg et al.'s study.

Some post-9/11 definitions have done a better job of accounting for the role of the witness in understanding the meanings and consequences of terrorism. Louise Richardson's definition of terrorism is particularly effective in considering witnesses as a crucial element in defining terrorism.[35] This definition sits within a tradition of describing terrorism through its constitutive elements rather than through one all encompassing and succinct statement.[36] This style for defining terrorism challenges the oversimplification and politicization of other, shorter definitions and therefore provides a broader, more complex and, I argue, more reliable context for understanding terrorism. Richardson herself does not claim to have even formulated a definition and identifies her efforts as "seven crucial characteristics of the term terrorism". Three of these account for the role of the witness.[37] These are: terrorism is a form of communication; terrorism has symbolism; and terrorism has victims and an audience. In relation to the first of these elements – terrorism as communication – Richardson argues that terrorism is not a nihilistic pursuit where violence represents an end in itself, nor is it aimed at defeating an enemy. Terrorist violence is designed as a message generator for an audience of witnesses.[38] The second element – the victims and violence are symbolic – Richardson argues: "The shock value of the act is enormously enhanced by the power of the symbol that the target represents". As such, terrorism works by creating a psychological impact greater than the "actual physical act" or the risks associated with the consequences of further terrorism.[39] The witness, in this view, perceives terrorism disproportionately to the danger it poses relative to other risks and dangers. Richardson is not alone in this claim. Horgan similarly argues that terrorism is designed to arouse witnesses to be threatened to a greater degree than the damage that terrorism will likely cause.[40] Friedland and Merari once argued that the perceptions of terrorism held by witnesses were worse than the act itself and allowed the affects of terrorism to be felt by people far beyond, both temporally and geographically, the initial destruction.[41] The third element that Richardson identifies that accounts for the role of the witness – terrorism has victims and an audience of witnesses – suggests that acts of terrorism are designed to affect the behavior of a group of people who witness the violence, not the behavior of those who die in an attack. Through the power of global images of terrorism captured by the news media and in screen cultures, such audiences of witnesses view terrorism in multiple configurations of time and space.

It is the creation of images and imagery that has afforded terrorists the power to reach audiences of witnesses far beyond the initial destruction of terrorist violence. Žižek argues that the 9/11 terrorists "did not do it primarily to provoke real material damage, but *for the spectacular effect of it*".[42] They were able to create what Weinmann and Winn described as the theater of terrorism. This theater is a place where violence is combined with images to create something greater than either violence or images alone.[43] From the beginning of the twentieth century terrorism was being increasingly described as theater as terrorists demonstrated their media savvy in their manipulation of governments, the press, witnesses, victims and images.[44] Anarchists that were operating in the early twentieth century were able to carry out high profile attacks that received media attention across the world, particularly in Europe and America. Their terrorism combined the intent to spread a message (propaganda) through the vessel of terrorism (the deed) in their strategy of generating terrifying and powerful images and imagery.[45] The anarchists quickly learned that the more spectacular the terrorism they staged, the more likely it was that the media and the public were paying attention. Whilst it may seem a little out of place in a discussion of terrorism, I argue the Vietnam War represented an important development in the history of image violence and witnessing terror. The Vietnam War brought terror and violence into the homes of people in many countries and its impact continues to resonate as images in the news media, popular, screen and tele-visual cultures. Fictional reanimations and re-imaginings of the Vietnam War have long been a cornerstone of screen cultures. Rick Berg has argued that this war characterized a generation, as 9/11 likely will.[46] For Berg, television "brought the war home" since "TV witnessed the event actually happening".[47]

Among the most powerful demonstrations of the ability of terrorists to attract audiences of witnesses by generating terrifying images occurred on 14 June 1985. A *TransWorld Airlines* (TWA) jet carrying 150 people was hijacked by a terrorist organization calling itself *Islamic Jihad*.[48] The plane was forced to fly between Athens, Beirut and Algiers and the world's media reported the events as they unfolded. People tuned in daily to watch and witness the terrorism spectacle unfold. The siege lasted 17 days. The most enduring images from this stand-off were created when a man was killed and thrown out of the plane in full view of news cameras. Images of this murder were beamed to news affiliates throughout the world and replayed on news programs and featured in newspapers. As a result, the media was heavily criticized, especially journalists from America, for providing terrorists with a platform to communicate their violent message. Rosen wrote in the *Wall Street Journal*: "Have (U.S) television journalists forgotten they are American? Everyone knows that terrorists want publicity for their cause, yet no less do they want to inflate their own personal status in their communities ... Therefore, each time the media afford the right to speak, they award them a victory!"[49] In response, the American journalist Tom Wicker wrote: "It may on occasion be inconvenient, intrusive, even harmful; but if because of government censorship or network censorship the hostage crisis had not been visible, *real*, on American screens, the outrage and outcry would have been a thousand times louder".[50] During the 17 day standoff, 491 hostage stories were reported on American television news amounting to 12 hours of real-time coverage.[51]

Whilst these moments of witnessing terrorism were indeed powerful, they remain less significant than the ultimate terrorism image-event that tele-visually unfolded in real-time on 9/11. This attack – what Jean Baudrillard described as the "mother" of all events[52] – generated a particularly powerful combination of violence and images and created something that is far more powerful and terrifying than violence or images alone. As Nacos argues, aside from the few who were alerted by friends and family via phone calls from the planes and buildings and those on the streets below the Towers, millions of people witnessed 9/11 via television news, radio broadcasts, and the Internet.[53] Michael Barnett writes of learning about the attacks from the television in his New York City apartment only a few miles from the World Trade Center.[54] Prominent cultural studies academic Toby Miller turned on the television even though the Twin Towers were burning close by.[55] Both were witnesses living and working in New York City, yet they joined distant audiences of witnesses in watching the continuous replays of the planes crashing into the Towers.

Researching Witnesses, Researching Screen Cultures

Whilst 9/11 was not the first act of terror to be re-imagined in televisual, popular and screen cultures, it has become the new referent for understanding the power of terror on the screen. It is the terror by which all terror past and future is understood. 9/11 has paved the way for an avalanche of popular and screen culture artifacts, some of which I will explore in detail in this book. This book is hardly the first attempt to account for post-9/11 popular culture. This trail has been blazed by others and I will explore their work in these pages. There has been a trend in this literature to be at once broader and more specific. Kristiaan Versluys, for example, explores at length post-9/11 novels and the role of storytelling in an age of terror.[56] By focussing on one medium, a certain critical depth is provided. Yet this depth comes at the expense of an analysis of other pop-cultural and screen cultural mediums. Stephen Prince explores post-9/11 films.[57] Again, specificity of medium comes at the expense of the broader perspective that would come from approaching pop-culture, screen culture and tele-visual culture as mining-sites for post-9/11 artifacts. Jeffrey Melnick's book 9/11 *Culture* achieves much to this end in his account of all things 9/11 in a post-9/11 world.[58]

I want to take this a step further. I want to focus in on particularly powerful post-9/11 moments in screen cultures rather than attempting to cover all aspects of 9/11 culture. To do this I will survey several fields of screen culture in various ways, with various methods. My focus will be on films, television, the blogosphere and the internet, fashion photography and the accounts of other witnesses of 9/11 and terrorism. In doing so, I encounter an overwhelming amount of information and data – what John Law would describe as social scientific "mess".[59] The methods for collecting and analyzing this mess see me sometimes occupying the guise of a sociologist, ethnographer, interviewer, narrative analyst, visual media interpreter, television and film watcher. Always as a witness. To these ends I am inspired by Law's arguments in favour of "method assemblage".[60]

> If new realities "out-there" and new knowledges of those realities "in-here" are to be created, then practices that can cope with a hinterland of pre-existing social and material realities also have to be built up and sustained. I call the enactment of this hinterland and its bundle of ramifying relations a "method assemblage".[61]

Method assemblages allow me to be many things at once and analyze many things in various ways. As such, this book sees me conduct and interpret qualitative interviews; interrogate the blogosphere; watch and theorize the meanings of television shows; explore when it might be possible to laugh at trauma; search for the illusive line between terrorism and pornography or at least show that one may not exist; and explore whether our imaginations have run wild. All with the aim of understanding the meanings and consequences of 9/11 and terrorism.

In doing so, I am a witness like many others, but I position myself as a special kind of witness in order to write this book. I am what Haraway would describe as a "modest witness" – a witness as social researcher.[62] In her critique of the modest witness Haraway wrote:

> He bears witness: he is objective; he guarantees the clarity and purity of objects. His subjectivity is his objectivity. His narratives have a magical power – they lose all trace of their history as stories, as products of partisan projects, as contestable representations, or as constructed documents in their potent capacity to define the facts.[63]

I follow Haraway in wanting to move away from this kind of modest witness and become a "more corporeal, inflected, and optically dense, if less elegant, kind of modest witness". I want to be critical of my witnessing, compare it with other moments of witnessing, but still bear witness myself, and write what I see. In my accounts of my witnessing I want to be involved in processes of "Interrogating critical silences, excavating the reasons questions cannot make headway and seem ridiculous, getting at the denied and disavowed in the heart of what seems neutral and rational".[64] My witnessing is situated, and I attempt to account for this situatedness as I proceed. This situatedness brings in other witnesses. I don't believe it is simply a matter of "I"; there is a "we" at stake in witnessing terrorism. The "we" is my assumption of what Law calls "out-thereness".[65] The "in-here" is the screen cultural moments that I have witnessed and that have expanded all of our capacities to witness terrorism. In short, I believe that millions of other people, perhaps more, are witnesses of terrorism just like me. I believe that others must have witnessed some of what I have witnessed in screen culture, a witnessing that I report on here in this book. But what are we witnessing in these "public and collective" moments?[66] Who are *we*?

A Sociology of "We"

The meanings and consequences of terrorism change with time. What is terrifying in one context may not be terrifying in another. Even as I write the meanings and consequences of terrorism are changing. Another terror attack in war-ravaged Iraq, this time to disrupt the 2010 elections. Another terrorist "mastermind" captured in Pakistan, but we have heard that before. Another conspiracy theory. And, perhaps inevitably, another devastating attack. Or, from the perspective of the global Westernized media, another devastating attack in a Western city. When I spoke to witnesses of 9/11 in the distant city of Melbourne, Australia in 2005 I was told that terrorism posed everyday problems for the inhabitants of this city. 9/11 had caused considerable terror and anxiety in a location that could hardly be further from the fire, smoke and debris being inhaled by New Yorkers on, and for weeks after, 9/11. When I casually talked with other witnesses of 9/11 in Melbourne in 2008 however, I received some quizzical looks and explanations that we know now that terrorism probably will not happen in Melbourne in the foreseeable future. Yet, many still feared terrorism and were permanently scarred by the tele-visual spectacle that they had witnessed on 9/11 and their sleepless night that followed (9/11 occurred in real-time late at night Australian time and the coverage continued round-the-clock throughout the night and for many days after the attacks). When I visit other cities in Australia and around the world I learn that terrorism was witnessed quite differently in different locations. I met a PhD student who was studying multiculturalism and whiteness in New Zealand; an understudied subject. When I asked whether the project had a post-9/11 context, I received a strange look and an "err, no".

Witnessing, in short, becomes differentiated across time and space. Witnesses, by their nature, are unstable and unpredictable. The word "witness" seeks to stabilize this instability. The witness is powerfully grounded in an event, in a location, in a moment in time. This makes the task of fashioning a stable language for talking about terrorism – a language that allows for both the changing and stable nature of the witness of terrorism to be explored – difficult as those who have attempted to define "terrorism" have discovered. The often heard cliché that one person's terrorist is another's freedom fighter is only one way to deal with this problem. It is a cliché that emphasizes the subjectivity of witnessing terrorism. But how do we describe and categorize witnesses and, in the process, create better witnesses? I suggest that there is an "us", or – even better – "we". It is a "we" that experiences *terror* when the debris and fire of an attack has settled. A "we" that debates where and when the next terror attack may occur. A "we" that wants swift justice against the perpetrators and terrorism's root causes challenged. Then there is another category of witness often described as "them" or "they". These people will belong to the racial, cultural, religious, political or ideological groups that the perpetrators of terror also belong to. Or perhaps "they" refers to those who do not oppose terrorism fervently enough, who are accused of being sympathetic to the terrorists' cause. In the present wave of terror, "they" and "them" have invariably been terms applied to Muslims, especially those living in diasporic communities. Sometimes it has involved picking a side in the "War on Terror" as former US President George W. Bush demonstrated when immediately after 9/11 he said that you are "either with us, or you are with the terrorists".

Or, stated differently, terror-talk inevitably invokes the language of *you, me, I, we, us* and *them*. In talking about terrorism some have taken great care to avoid this language, whilst others have embraced it. This language is important. It may decide who is a terrorist and who is merely a "militant", "guerilla" or an "insurgent". Who violently opposes terrorism and who holds sympathies. As Noam Chomsky has argued, terrorism for too long has been defined as the crimes that "*they* carry out against us", whoever *we* happen to be.[67] Manning has argued that the news media after 9/11 was quick to frame terrorism as a problem of "Us and Them".[68] Yet shedding such terms in discussing terrorism is perhaps not as easy as it may seem. Some drop away easily. Instead of saying "them" or "they" we can perhaps be more specific. It is perhaps a problem of "Islamic extremism" or the more insulting "Islamo-fascism". Perhaps we can emphasize geographical dimensions. The terrorists were "Egyptian", "Saudi", or "Pakistani". In the present wave of terror these commonly used terms do little to undermine the myth that Muslims are intrinsically linked to terrorism, but they at least open a space where alternative phrasing can be used. Terrorists may be Hindu-extremists, Christian-extremists, Irish radicals, anti-state or anti-globalization revolutionaries, home-grown and so on. "They" and "them" can be easily discarded with an appeal to specificity. I have found "I", "Us" and "We" to be far more stubborn. "We" indicates that the speaker is part of a group, the same group that the speaker is addressing. It treats an indefinite number of people as a generalizable mass which, in most instances, is not desirable in scholarly endeavors. But 9/11 is not an ordinary event, and its consequences betray normality. It has proved difficult for me to find someone not touched by the consequences of 9/11, someone who does not – in one way or another – fit within this "we"; the audiences of witnesses of 9/11. In any exploration of the meanings and consequences of terrorism this stubborn "we" must be accounted for since I have found its use to be unavoidable.

This book is, in part, an attempt to account for this "we" in understanding the meanings and consequences of terrorism and the meanings and consequences of social science research. Social scientists must assume that there is an emergent and contextual "we" from time to time, even as they acknowledge that this "we" is far from being an unproblematic construct. "We" in this book is a tool, a resource, and a means to an end. It is a "we" that positions the witness as the innocent and blameless victim of terrorism. At the same time the picture is more complex than this. "We" is perhaps an essential coordinate for understanding what it means to witness violent, spectacular events like 9/11 and terrorism, and for living with the consequences of violent image-events in times of terror.

When I use the word "we" in this book I do so deliberately and with full awareness of its problematic nature – it generalizes unique individuals, each with a story to tell, as eye-witnesses of 9/11. As such, it is a mythical and chimeric construct, a made-up creation of a social scientist's mind. This "we", which is an attempt to account for large numbers of people, may account for no-one at all. Yet, in many respects, I do intend to imply an undifferentiated "we". I am talking about a particular "we". The "we" that were the witnesses in the audiences of the global theater of terror. This "we" share much in common. *We* witnessed 9/11. For many of us, we witnessed 9/11 as a real-time event as the Towers fell. And *we* have witnessed 9/11's startling and sometimes absurd consequences. *We* have witnessed two international wars fought in its name. *We* have witnessed so-called enemy combatants captured in these theaters and exported to Cuba where they have been "interrogated" and made subject to "rendition" (spin-doctoring for merciless torture). In a bizarre twist, *we* witnessed torture first-hand through images that emerged from the notorious (under both Saddam and US occupation) Abu Ghraib prison in Iraq. Not only were "enemy combatants" tortured in this prison, but the torture was captured on digital cameras, complete with US military personnel moronically grinning, seemingly proud with their obscene torture, seemingly unaware that the sexualized violence cast doubt on the US war effort, its purpose and appropriateness (I explore these images further in chapter seven). *We* also witnessed as fear and anxiety permeated cities throughout the world. *We* have witnessed Muslims targeted for the way they look as much as for their religious beliefs and their perceived links to terrorism (importantly, *looking* Muslim was far more important than being Muslim).

But what exactly, precisely, did we witness?

First, there was the ultimate event, the "mother" of all events,[69] a real-world event and an image-event; "Ground Zero". The post-9/11 world *feels* a certain way. It has certain dimensions and contours. It is a world of renewed war-waging, war-spending and war-fetishism. The mother of all events set the tone for a post-9/11 world filled with terror scares, near-misses and front page terror-gossip. Who has captured who? Who has threatened to bomb who? Who are the most guilty? Are the US imperialists or are terrorists freedom haters? The 9/11 attacks worked to both forge this "we" and to simultaneously differentiate it. We were all witnesses, but we witnessed in different ways, in different places, at different times. I was in my bedroom in my family's home in a provincial town resting between two major cities in Australia. I stayed up all night watching the coverage (which was round-the-clock on all of Australia's free-to-air television networks), occasionally stopping to make a coffee or to call friends to make sure they were watching. The next day, I attended the university where I was an undergraduate. 9/11 was the only topic of conversation. In my classes, every academic wanted to talk about 9/11. My economics professor made the class destroy the economy and rebuild it using only economics.[70]

The round-the-clock coverage continued for many days. Then we witnessed the tributes, the pain and the sorrow as what had just happened began to sink in. All the while, television cameras captured the images. It was a spectacle like no other. 9/11 was spectacular. The sorrow was spectacular. The tributes were spectacular. And the ferocious US reprisals in Afghanistan and Iraq were spectacular. The spectacle, by its nature, is excessive. The study of the spectacle of terrorism is becoming an important field of post-9/11 theory and research.[71] As such, I do not offer a definition of terrorism for this book. Instead I offer a definition of *terrorism as spectacle* in order to fuse the power of 9/11 as a global event with the power of 9/11 as a global image-event. I define *terrorism as spectacle* as the use of terrorism in ways that translate readily into terrifying mediated images: into terrifying symbolic events. In doing so, such events can be viewed and consumed by global audiences of witnesses. These witnesses occupy diverse configurations of time and space. Often these witnesses are not in close geographic proximity to the flashpoint of terrorist violence. Terrorism as spectacle seeks the largest audience possible. The spectacle terrorist plans to combine violence with image production to create something more powerful than the violence alone.[72]

With this definition I stress that terrorists have long known that one dead enemy in a cosmopolitan city is worth 100 in a war zone. It brings to the foreground the image and the witness for understanding terrorism and how the interactions between terrorism, tele-visual and screen cultures and witnesses has afforded terrorists a terrible power to spread fear and anxiety to distant corners of the planet.

Through the power of this spectacle the image-event on 9/11 paved the way for other image-events as 9/11 entered not only our imaginations, but began to saturate our popular culture. As regular viewing began to resume after 9/11 we witnessed television programs that were set in New York City change. No longer did the Twin Towers feature in their rolls of stock footage that structured opening and closing credits and transitions between scenes (I explore this in some depth in chapter four). Then we witnessed the feature films and the television portrayals of terrorism and 9/11. We witnessed Jack Bauer fight terrorists in real time on *24*,[73] Jennifer Garner demonstrate spy chic in *Alias*,[74] and *United 93*[75] and *World Trade Center*[76] took American anti-terror cheerleading to a new level. This cheerleading was countered by conspiracy theorists who believe that 9/11 was staged by the US government and others who questioned the US government's actions before and after 9/11. Movies such as *Loose Change*[77] and *Fahrenheit 9/11*[78] became signposts in a 9/11 counterculture that disputed a number of the accepted facts reported about 9/11. Documentaries, news programs, religious ministers, teams of academics and experts, and government spokespeople and diplomats all weighed into the debate about 9/11 and its meanings and consequences. Opinion columnists and "shock jocks" fashioned debates on the merits of bombing civilian populations, detaining innocent people and the difference between wholesale torture or mere rendition and coercive interrogation. Television shows and films have continued to depict various aspects of the post-9/11 world. As the material, often murderous, consequences of 9/11 endure, so too have images of 9/11. In many ways, they have become a routine and ordinary – yet ambiguous and ambivalent – part of life.

Allegory and Witnessing Terrorism

The everydayness of terrorism, and its ambiguous and ambivalent nature, is a fertile ground from which post-9/11 *allegory* has emerged. Allegory in witnessing terrorism is a central and reoccurring theme in this book. For John Law allegory "is the art of meaning something other and more than what is being said … it is the art of decoding that meaning, reading between the literal lines to understand what is actually being depicted".[79] Engaging with post-9/11 allegory – and its brethren irony, trope and metaphor – in terrorism studies is the path less traveled; it is like standing on the wrong building. The study of post-9/11 allegory is, for the most part, of little interest to those whose job it is to prevent and mitigate the consequences of terrorism (government officials, some academics, security and intelligence personnel, the police and the military). However, for witnesses of 9/11 and terrorism, it is a familiar occurrence. The framing of terrorism in popular, tele-visual and screen cultures is designed for these witnesses. Their ability to read "between the literal lines" makes them experts in understanding the meanings and consequences of spectacular images of terrorism.

Allegory, it would seem, is closely related to images. In allegorical moments the "*appearance* of direct representation is the effect of a process of artful deletion".[80] Even as 9/11 was occurring as images of horrific violence, it was concealing. It was *Othering*. Among that which was Othered in the spectacular images of 9/11 was a sense of why it was happening, how it had been permitted to occur. It Othered a legacy of violence perpetrated by successive US governments in the years leading up to 9/11. It Othered generations of oppression experienced by the hijackers. It Othered the lack of co-ordination of US law enforcement and intelligence authorities. And it Othered the ferocious US reprisals that were to come. These Others, and many other Others, were drowned out by the immediate brutality of the spectacular and obscene violence and destruction. But, as the dust settled, spaces opened for Others to return. Many returned as allegory.

Indeed, many who acknowledged these Others too soon after 9/11 were accused of standing on the wrong building, even of having misplaced ideas of the world and the meaning of terrorism. But it was not long before these Others also became routine, yet ambivalent and ambiguous, features of the post-9/11 world.

Post-9/11 popular, tele-visual and screen cultures have played a crucial role in representing 9/11 as allegory. The creators and producers of these cultures used "what is present as a resource to mess about with absence", make "manifest what is otherwise invisible", and extend "the fields of visibility" to produce "new realities".[81] Allegory, stated differently, "makes space for *ambivalence and ambiguity*".[82] Allegory allows for previously Othered realities to become manifest, but often in partial, fractured and "non-coherent" ways.[83] Reality, images, allegory, fiction – there is something missing, something obviously absent, in this equation. The missing figure is the witness, the audience. Witnesses of terrorism in reality, in images, in allegory, in fiction.

How This Book is Structured

This book is in two parts – part one (chapters one, two and three) is designed to set the stage. It is designed to lay the foundations for understanding how terrorism is witnessed, spectacularized, interpreted and remembered and how this is the beginning of a journey that ends with *terror on the screen*. The witnesses of terrorism are brought to the foreground in my attempt to understand the meanings and consequences of terrorism. Indeed, witnesses have always been critical in successful terrorist attacks although this has seldom been acknowledged in the terrorism studies literature. The witness has traditionally been *Othered* – made absent in the pursuit of the perpetrators of terrorism and the enhancement of security to prevent further attacks.

In chapter two I explore what it means to live in the terrorists' visual playground – the contemporary city. Following Baudrillard, Žižek and the film *The Matrix*, I argue, with a strong sense of the allegorical, that the city is a *desert of the real* – a place that possesses all of the props and actors for the theater of terrorism. It is a place where reality is laid bare and where Hollywood disaster films enter *reality*. I report on interviews that were conducted in one theater of the desert of the real and, in doing so, share the stories of witnesses of 9/11 and terrorism, witnesses that found themselves caught in the cross-hairs as contemporary terrorists' targets of choice.

In the third chapter I examine the meanings of *celebrity terrorism*. Terrorism and celebrity cultures have much in common and share many of the same spaces and the terrorism studies literature has important cross-over points with the celebrity culture literature. I explore these literatures and interrogate some of these cross-over points by exploring moments when terrorism filled the blogosphere and other online spaces. These blogs and internet spaces provide situated insights into post-9/11 cultures of witnessing terrorism.

Part two of this book (chapters four, five, six and seven) provides critical explorations of various fields of popular, tele-visual and screen cultures through which 9/11 is witnessed, spectacularized, interpreted and remembered. These chapters are, in many respects, case studies – working examples of post-9/11 witnessing, allegory and remembering at work.

Chapter four presents post-9/11 episodes of the popular television program *Friends*. They are special artifacts of post-9/11 screen culture. In these episodes there was, in some respects, a response to 9/11 based in silence and absences. Yet, paradoxically, 9/11 was still present as a kind of traumatic echo. Through various references to 9/11 and post-9/11 culture, *Friends* paid tribute to 9/11. Yet there was no role for 9/11 in the narrative of post-9/11 *Friends*. It was as though terrorism had never occurred in the New York City of these six friends going about their everyday lives in Manhattan. This presence-absence of 9/11 in post-9/11 *Friends* embodies a traumatic reaction, a reaction that seeks to disavow 9/11 in the face of its obvious horror and tragedy.

The fifth chapter offers accounts of the post-9/11 episodes of another popular television show; the re-imagined *Battlestar Galactica* (BSG). This program was designed for the post-9/11 consumer. It contains many themes and narratives that offer insight and commentary on why 9/11 occurred and the subsequent "War on Terror". The re-imagined BSG reminds us that when history repeats and traumatic events occur as a consequence, they do so *the first time as tragedy, the second time as farce*. BSG is a cautionary tale for a post-9/11 world in which the next 9/11 may be just around the corner. As long as wars are waged and people are oppressed, it is likely that counter-movements will rise to confront the oppressor.

In chapter six I pursue post-9/11 narratives of comedy/trauma in television and film. This chapter is designed to highlight these narratives in a way that demonstrates how post-9/11 comedy and trauma are deeply related. The chapter's first half features narratives of trauma, the chapter's second half features narratives of comedy. With these oppositional but deeply connected narratives I show that comedy and trauma are kin. Trauma can easily give way to comedy, and comedy can give way to trauma. Television shows such as *The Simpsons*, John Stewart's *The Daily Show*, *American Dad* and *Family Guy*, and movies like *Team America: World Police*, rely on this kinship. When we laugh at trauma it need not cause more pain and disrespect. It can be a cathartic moment and a moment for patriotic unity.

In the seventh chapter I explore the strange but powerful links between terrorism and pornography – a fusion that I call *Terrorsex*.

I argue that terrorsex can be found in some unlikely places and can emerge in some unlikely ways. When the image, the spectacle and the *witness as voyeur* emerge as privileged sites for understanding terrorism, terrorsex is the likely outcome. I analyze some crucial moments of terrorsex – a fashion shoot in *Vogue: Italia* magazine titled "State of Emergency", the television show *Dollhouse*, and the disturbing images of sexual abuse of prisoners in Abu Ghraib prison in Iraq. It has often been said that terrorism is like pornography, that we know it when we see it. But terrorsex threatens to undermine any clear distinctions between pornography and terror by offering a commodified fusion of terror and porn in some unlikely spaces.

The final chapter sees me build on Noam Chomsky's notion of a "Culture of Terrorism". In a post-9/11 world, this culture exists but as something different to what Chomsky imagined. The post-9/11 world is characterized by what I call a *screen culture of terrorism*. The screen culture of terrorism distorts our visions as witnesses of 9/11 and overwhelms us with excesses of terrorism and violence. This terror and violence has also overwhelmed our imaginations. In this way, terrorists have targeted us where we are most vulnerable and least able to resist. Screen cultures of terrorism have infiltrated our lives in routine and banal ways and, in doing so, have disrupted what it means to live in the "everyday" as precarious and vulnerable witnesses of terrorism. The screen culture of terrorism is *our* culture, and it is a culture where our imaginations have run wild.

Conclusion

While standing on the red carpet for the 2010 Oscars, the star of the film *Precious* – Gabourey Sidibe – said: "If fashion was porn, this dress would be the money shot".[84] The moment that the second airplane struck Tower Two on 9/11 can be seen as a metaphorical "money shot".[85] The moment that grabs our attention, the moment that forces us to witness, unable to look away despite our pain, disbelief, fear and disgust. This money shot is responsible for the groundswell of post-9/11 screen culture and our cultural obsession with terrorism. Journalists and newspaper editors have long known that terrorism, like sex, sells. Since 9/11, creators, producers and writers of screen culture have realized this too (although I am

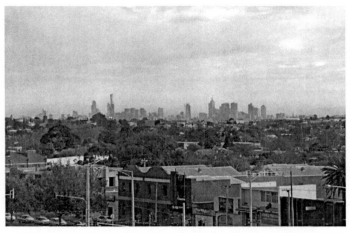

View of Melbourne from Monash University, Caulfield

certain they have long known this, but what they perhaps lacked was the tele-visual "money shot" that 9/11 provided).

On the occasion of the 7th anniversary of 9/11 I was participating in a reading group hosted by my colleagues at Monash University in suburban Melbourne, Australia. Reading groups such as these occurred from time to time, usually in the picturesque fifth level common room of a recently built ten-story building on Monash University's Caulfield campus located about 10 kilometers (just over six miles) from Melbourne's city center. The large windows in this room offer views of Australian suburbia, Port Phillip Bay and the attractive Melbourne skyline. On this day, we all admired these views from time to time as we discussed the reading we were studying. In all, it was a routine Melbourne day.

Without needing to say anything we were all suddenly aware of a glitch in our view of suburbia, bay and city. There was a small object – a passenger airplane, perhaps a "747" – flying in close proximity to the Melbourne skyline. We were briefly transfixed on this object. We watched and we witnessed. We witnessed the plane move closer to the Melbourne skyline, we witnessed the plane disappear, we witnessed the plane re-appear on the other side of our view of the Melbourne skyline and continue on its way to a domestic destination or perhaps Singapore, LAX, London or some other international locale. This was a part of my 9/11, circa. 2008.

Our harmless encounter with this plane represented a simple routine, yet from our location we could not help but recognize the image, the scene, the theater. Planes fly near and around cities throughout the world frequently. But it was the image of a plane next to the city skyline that struck us all. It was an image that we had seen before on that day seven years earlier. Images of terrorism work that way. They stick with witnesses, bundled up with the trauma of terrorism. It was a traumatic flashback that made us all watch, just for a moment, before we all returned to our conversation.

Then US President, George W. Bush, addressed the American people on this same anniversary through the usual globally net-worked, tele-visual channels. He described 9/11 as the "worst day in America's history" but it was also a day for "some of the bravest acts" Americans had ever performed.[86] In Manhattan, thousands of people from over 90 countries came together to hear the famous 9/11 "roll call" that commemorates the 2751 people that were known to have died in the coordinated attacks in that location on that day.[87] The Whitehouse Press Secretary, Dana Perino, said that "The president thinks about 9/11 every single day when he wakes up and before he goes to bed".[88] There have been many moments like these since the 11 September 2001 terrorist attacks. Thinking about 9/11 is not something reserved for the former President. Many people, living and working in many different places throughout the world have had first-hand experience with terrorism, whether they witnessed terrorism live on the streets of their city, or in a city far away. What many near and distant witnesses have in common is that they witnessed terrorism not as debris and shrapnel falling around them with the heat of the flames singeing their face. Rather, many both near and far from where terrorism has occurred have witnessed terrorism as a tele-visual mediated event, as an artifact of screen culture, as a globalized image-event. Witnessing terrorism in such a way does little to curb its terrifying consequences.

As witnesses, we have been nurtured in the post-9/11 world. When our televisions, cinemas and the internet turn us into terror-voyeurs I do not believe that we can simply blame the 9/11 hijackers. We must take some responsibility. 9/11 entered the world fixed in the time and space coordinates of 11 September 2001 in New York, Washington DC and a field in Pennsylvania. But it has been able to exploit the complex conditions of the post-9/11 world to transcend these coordinates. It remains that the tele-visual, popular and screen cultures that I explore in this book are products made possible *post*-9/11, not by 9/11 itself. This makes this book quite different to others that have tackled this topic. After all, *9/11 itself* plays little role in the cultures I explore in this book. A cartoon about a CIA agent – called *American Dad* – was possible pre-9/11, but has new meaning post-9/11. *Friends* existed before 9/11, and had new meaning after 9/11. *Battlestar Galactica* existed in one form before 9/11, and was *re-imagined* after 9/11. Josh Whedon made most of *Buffy* and *Angel* before 9/11, but *Dollhouse* after 9/11.

Where the amorphous threat of terrorism meets its intended audience, the witnesses of terrorism, the spectacle reigns. The arguments, theories and case studies contained in this book are designed to shift the focus for understanding the meanings and consequences of terrorism away from more traditional fields of terrorism and counterterrorism research such as the psychology of terrorists; the prevention and mitigation of terrorism through the development of technical security systems; risk management; the study of biological, radiological, chemical and nuclear threats; war and insurgency; the morality and philosophy of terrorism; ideology and politics; diasporic communities; medical capabilities and responses; counterterrorism policing; and a host of other related fields spread across social and natural sciences and academic, security, intelligence, diplomatic and political communities and groups. *I think they have that covered.* I want to redirect attention towards what I argue to be the most important method for understanding terrorism – *witnessing*. Without witnessing, there would be no emotional response to label *terror*. There would be dead bodies, and ruined buildings and infrastructure, but if no one sees it, surely it cannot be called terrorism. *If a terrorist fells a tree in the woods, would the media report it?* Witnessing terrorism involves images, spectacles and a vantage point. 9/11 holds power as an image-event because that vantage point may have been anywhere across the world. There were few barriers to eye-witnessing on 9/11 as real-time feeds from Manhattan filled the screens of audiences of witnesses in the global theater of terrorism.

2.

Welcome to the City, Welcome to the Desert of the Real

I remember … remarking on the criminal futility of the whole thing, doctrine, action, mentality; and on the contemptible aspect of the half-crazy pose as of a brazen cheat exploiting the poignant miseries and passionate credulities of a mankind always so tragically eager for self-destruction … Presently, passing to particular instances, we recalled the already old story of the attempt to blow up the Greenwich Observatory; a blood-stained inanity of so fatuous a kind that it was impossible to fathom its origin by any reasonable process of thought. For *perverse unreason* has its own logical processes.[1]

In the previous chapter I emphasized the role of witnessing in understanding the meanings and consequences of terrorism and the ways in which terrorism is spectacularized, interpreted and remembered. I emphasized how witnessing has always been an important, but mostly absent, feature for understanding terrorism; what I mean when I use the word "we"; and the significance of popular, tele-visual and screen cultures in bringing terrorism into the realm of impression and the everyday. In this chapter I further some of these claims by exploring the spaces and locations where contemporary terrorism matters most. These spaces are located *in the city*. While it is often argued that terrorism targets innocents, civilians and noncombatants, it is rarely acknowledged that terrorists are far more selective than this in choosing their victims. Victims must not only be innocent, non-military and noncombatant; they must be symbolic and representative of a broader audience of witnesses. Those who die or are injured in a terrorist attack are never arbitrary or random targets – they are carefully selected to make an audience of witnesses *terrified*.

9/11 is a powerful example of terrorist logics at work – the terrorists' *"perverse unreason"*. I have heard media commentators suggest that 9/11 was random and arbitrary violence, but this is clearly wrong. The Twin Towers and the workers within were a powerful symbol of US economic hegemony, and the Pentagon and its political, intelligence and military staff were powerful symbols of US military hegemony. The plane that crashed in Pennsylvania was said to be heading to Washington DC, perhaps to the Whitehouse – yet another symbolic target, the equivalent of a "decapitation attack" (although the President was not there at the time). These targets were hardly chosen by irrational psychopaths. These were calculated choices. They were targets that were designed to not only strike a devastating blow to the US's economic, military or political power – an attack with such a far-reaching goal would undoubtedly fail. The United States, like any country, is made of more than its parts. Rather, the devastating blows on 9/11 were designed to undermine emotional, psychological, social and cultural well-being. They were designed to cause fear and spread terror. They were designed to illicit an obscene and excessive response that would delegitimize the US throughout the world. But Americans were not the only ones who felt terror on 9/11. Global audiences of tele-visual witnesses became consumed by the attacks, and the denizens of cities throughout the world began to wonder where the terrorists would strike next. These witnesses examined their own cities for security flaws. Our buildings are tall and symbolic, we have intricate and heavily relied upon public transport systems, we have government buildings. *We could be next!*

I put this idea to the test in a city that could hardly be further removed from Manhattan, Washington DC, or even Pennsylvania. The city I chose was my city, a city that had never experienced a significant and symbolic act of terrorism. Indeed people in my city had little reason to believe that terrorism would occur at any time. But 9/11 had left its scars. When I interviewed people that were living and working in this city in 2005, I discovered that fear and terror permeated the lives of city dwelling witnesses, even those far removed from the global violence raging in distant locations. They were distant witnesses, but distance has done little to diminish the power of 9/11.

Terrorism, the City and the Real

The title for this chapter was drawn from three related, yet distinct, sources. The first source was the blockbuster Wachowski brothers' film, *The Matrix*.[2] This film, among other things, tells the story of Thomas Anderson, also known as "Neo", and the world in which he lived. To Neo, this world had never felt quite right. It was a world that did not feel *real*. In his quest to learn more about this world he encounters the mysterious Trinity and Morpheus and he is given a choice – take the blue pill and go back to life as normal or take the red pill and discover how unreal the world truly is. Neo takes the red pill and undergoes a traumatic transformation, awaking into the *real* world. What Neo learns is that the world he had been living in – the Matrix – was a tele-visual, simulated wonderland that presented itself as everything he saw, heard, felt, smelled and touched. In reality every human brain was plugged into a super-computer that simulated the world, beaming images directly into their minds generating an illusion that occupied the minds and bodies of the human slaves. The film represented dichotomies of reality: illusion and real; fake and authentic; present and future. In this paradoxically simultaneous present/future/fake/authentic visual reality – the world around us, the world inside the Matrix – was the present, whereas the hidden world – the world of the real, outside the Matrix – resided in the future. Inside the Matrix humankind is, "in reality", plugged-in to a machine as the battery-power for a virtual world of human existence: the very world we see around us. The world outside of the Matrix is a post-apocalyptic wasteland. In one of the film's epic and most well known scenes, Neo is wrenched out of the Matrix and awakened to the desolate wasteland of the "future". Morpheus, the resistance leader who frees Neo, introduced this world to him with the ironic phrase: "*Welcome to the desert of the real!*"[3]

The second source for the title of this chapter is Jean Baudrillard's work in *Simulacra and Simulation*.[4] He argued in this book that the simulation – what he called hyperreality – is far more real than reality itself. Baudrillard described what he meant by this with reference to an old tale of a cartographer who made a map of an Empire so detailed and so precise that it covered the entire Empire – the Empire was entirely simulated as a map.[5] Baudrillard argued that in contemporary times, times that are defined and understood through glossy media imagery that simulates real events, it is the edges of reality that are fraying, not the edges of the map. As Baudrillard argued: "It is the real, and not the map, whose vestiges persist here and there in the deserts that are no longer those of the Empire, but ours. *The desert of the real itself*".[6]

The third source for the title of this chapter is Slavoj Žižek's post-9/11 book titled *Welcome to the Desert of the Real!*.[7] In this book Žižek argues that the 9/11 terrorist attacks have allowed witnesses to experience, once again, a "passion for the real".[8] It was the terrorists that awakened this passion and staged their destructive violence not only for the death and destruction it would cause but *"for the spectacular effect of it"*.[9]

These three sources are not mutually exclusive. Baudrillard's book was an inspiration to the Wachowski brothers and a guiding influence as they wrote *The Matrix*. In one scene from the film, Neo opened a copy of *Simulacra and Simulation*. The book had been hollowed out, and inside Neo stored some computer disks containing illegal programs that would presumably be used for hacking and other computer crimes. Indeed, Žižek in his account of the 9/11 attacks was making reference to *The Matrix* in his choice of title. These conceptualizations of the notion of the *desert of the real* all offer ways of exploring the meanings and consequences of the 9/11 terrorist attacks. This phrase is a metaphor for what occurred on 9/11 and how it was witnessed across the world via the global news media and for how these witnesses continued to live and work in cities that were indefinitely defined as *post*-9/11.

Images of Terrorism

Many witnesses viewed 9/11 through images transmitted to many distant locations even as it was occurring. For many distant (and nearby) witnesses 9/11 was a moving picture on a screen. But one of 9/11's most striking features is that whilst in reality it occurred in New York City (and Washington D.C. and Shanksville, Pennsylvania – but from a screen culture perspective, mainly in NYC), it also occurred in a series of symbolic locations. Whilst 9/11 certainly occurred in NYC, it also can be said to have occurred on television, in the city, in high rise buildings, in corporate offices, in government buildings, on the internet, replayed in the news media, and replayed as flashbacks in the minds of witnesses both near and far from the flames, death and destruction. Indeed, this is the nature and purpose of terrorism – to have a lot of people watching, not just a lot of people dead.[10] Terrorists want witnesses to toil in an anxious world where the next terror attack could seemingly come at any time, in any place. Terrorists want witnesses to toil in "the desert of the real".

In the desert of the real there is little certainty of security, an acute awareness of human vulnerability and precariousness, and the institutions that fashion and sustain existence are fractured and disorganized. The desert of the real can be any post catastrophe city. This city can be seen in Hollywood disaster movies such as *The Matrix*. It can also be seen in the footage of passenger airplanes being crashed into the Twin Towers. Consider for a moment a fundamental proposition in psychological studies literature of the function of the senses. In particular, consider the so-called visual association area of the brain. In this view, the eyes are neutral organs. They transmit stimuli that they do not understand to a part of the brain where visual interpretation occurs. Indeed, it is the brain that we can say truly does the *seeing*.[11] How then are we to distinguish between the real and the really real if it is little more than a matter of association, a matter of considering the new information in light of information that we already possess? How does the witness distinguish between what is an image of fictitious violence and what is an image of real violence?

> For the great majority of the public, the WTC explosions were events on the TV screen, and when we watched the oft-repeated shot of frightened people running towards the camera ahead of the giant cloud of dust from the collapsing tower, was not the framing of the shot itself reminiscent

of spectacular shots in catastrophe movies, a special effect which outdid all others, since ... reality is the best appearance of itself.[12]

The implication here is that fiction and reality are not easily distinguishable when they are both images. Baudrillard argued that on 9/11 the real absorbed the energy of fiction.[13] This is perhaps why some changed the channels on their televisions so they could be sure that 9/11 was really happening.[14] The images were comparable to those in catastrophe movies with one notable exception: 9/11 was real. Baudrillard argued that "the fascination with the attack is primarily a fascination with the image (both their exultatory and its catastrophic consequences are themselves largely imaginary)".[15]

Baudrillard argued that before 9/11 events were on strike, but the attacks on the World Trade Center represented an end of the strike.[16] 9/11 is the mother of all events, "the pure event uniting within itself all the events that have never taken place" – and it took place in the contemporary city. Indeed, the world's most recognizable city. When Baudrillard argued that 9/11 never took place he was not claiming that the terrorism on 9/11 was a cover-up or a conspiracy, that the attacks literally never took place, or that the Twin Towers are still standing. Rather, he was arguing that what has come to be relied upon as information and meaning does not convey the events only as a violent act, but also as an image. Without going to New York City, visiting Ground Zero, and seeing the hole in the ground, witnesses to the images of 9/11 can never verify that the Towers are gone. Witnesses, however, accept that the Towers are gone: it is an unwavering faith in images. Žižek posits the problem as a continuation of a trend where the "product is deprived of its substance" but retains a "hard resistant kernel of the real".[17] In this way 9/11 is one in a series of commodities that embody an absence: things that are "deprived of their malignant properties".[18] Milk and cream without fat, beer and spirits without alcohol (think of the "Claytons" drink: the drink you have when you are not having a drink), cakes and biscuits without sugar, coffee without caffeine, cyber-sex as sex without sex, Internet communities as societies without human contact, war without casualties, and multiculturalism as Others without their Otherness.

Witnesses in many cities throughout the world never viewed 9/11 as a *real* event.[19] It was terrorism as an image. Obscenely, it was violence without violence. Only a small percentage of 9/11's witnesses watched the violence as a *really* real event. The vast majority witnessed the event as *hyperreality* through images. But it was because 9/11 was a hyperreal event, an event captured and disseminated as a spectacular image, that it reached so many witnesses, many in other cities throughout the world.

One such city was the large multicultural city of Melbourne, Australia. I have conducted research in this city in which I interviewed people about how 9/11 has had meanings and consequences for their lives in this distant location. I report on this research later in this chapter. But for the moment, I want to further the argument that images of terrorism have special consequences in cityscapes. The result of this may be that all cities throughout the world are post-9/11 *traumascapes*.

Traumascapes

A *traumascape* is a location, a geographically defined space, that is infused with memories and histories of trauma.[20] They are locations that are known more for their violent and traumatic past than for their prosperous present or hopeful future. Traumascapes are solemn, emotional, and regretful places. People who visit or live and work in these locations are said to be touched and humbled by the histories and memories and by the resilience of the people who dwell there. Following Tumarkin I argue that post-9/11 cities – filled with vulnerable and precarious humans pursuing careers, life and leisure – can be viewed as *traumascapes*. Tumarkin argues that locations and spaces that have been the site for a disaster, a tragedy, or an act of destructive violence are forever imprinted with the memory of that event:

> *Traumascape* is not another, catchier, word for a site of tragedy, because "trauma" itself is not another word for tragedy or disaster ... It has a distinct meaning ... The word's continuous misuse obscures the fact that "traumatic" is in no way a synonym for "unpleasant" or "emotionally taxing" or even "intensely painful". One word that perhaps most

closely comes to expressing its meaning is "overwhelming".
A traumatised person cannot fully take in or comprehend
what has happened to them or what they have happened
to witness. They are *overwhelmed* by a traumatic event. So
much so that the ways in which they usually experience the
world and make sense of their own place in it are effectively
shattered.[21]

Tumarkin's study focuses directly on locations that have experienced horrific and spectacular violence; the physical places where
violence *happened* and the impact of that violence in that place
across time. Yet, every explanation of traumascape that Tumarkin
offers opens a space for an analysis of not only physical locations
of violence but also symbolic locations of violence, locations that
extend well beyond geographically defined boundaries of one city
or state or country. The contemporary city can be seen as one such
symbolic location that exists in a post-9/11 world. The 9/11 terrorist
attacks may have happened in NYC and Washington DC, but it is
clear that the consequences of these attacks – and all terrorist attacks – extend well beyond these locations. Through the power of
globally disseminated images of terrorism, post-9/11 traumascapes
can be found in cities throughout the world: "Because trauma is
contained not in an event as such but in the way this event is experienced, traumascapes become much more than physical settings
of tragedies: they emerge as spaces, where events are experienced
and re-experienced across time".[22] As such, traumascapes like the
contemporary city – a place where the seemingly constant threat of
terrorism is grappled with and negotiated in everyday and routine
ways – are full of "visual and sensory triggers" that are "capable of
eliciting a whole palette of emotions".[23] Or, stated differently, the
contemporary city contains all of the actors, scenery and special effects for a theater of terrorism.

For Bryan Turner, the vulnerability and precariousness of the
human body is both a product and a reflection of the vulnerability
and precariousness of the societies and institutions that structure
day-to-day human existence. Bauman has similarly suggested that
precariousness and vulnerability are unavoidable consequences of
life in the city.[24] The institutions and infrastructures that are found

in the city develop in response to human vulnerability yet, perhaps ironically, they exhibit many of the same vulnerabilities. In short, our quest for security improves our awareness that complete security is not possible. Or, when we believe we have found effective and complete security, we believe a myth, an image, a chimera, a simulation. The vulnerability of city spaces was a principle concern for Simmel when he argued that people acting socially were "dependent on the complementary activity of others".[25] Simmel argued that the institutions that organize and sustain human existence and their day-to-day lives are indispensable supports – both mentally and physically – for life in the city.[26] When these institutions are challenged, interrupted, de-routinized and violently disturbed, as they were on 9/11, it poses physical, psychological and emotional challenges to the everydayness of city living. This was perhaps one of the most shocking consequences of 9/11, the way New York City ceased to function in routine and everyday ways. This was something that New Yorkers shared with people in Iraqi cities after the US invasion. As Zillah Eisenstein writes of Iraq, post-invasion:

> Riverbend, the young Iraqi woman writing a daily blog, describes the dreariness of everyday life in war. She writes about the lack of electricity and water, about the unrelenting heat, and the night-time raids which meant people went to bed in their clothes, and the shortages of gasoline and its high cost. She writes of the daily life that doesn't happen, the daily routines that no longer exist. War is not just about dying; it is about living a life that isn't worth living.[27]

In chapter four of this book, I explore the meanings of everyday routines after 9/11 as they are represented in the popular television show *Friends*. Much like it did for Riverbend, the post-9/11 world ushered in for Americans a time when routines were ill defined and unreliable.[28] Fromm has argued that our routines play a vital role in living healthy psychological and emotional lives.[29] The ease with which terrorists have been able to disrupt these routines is one of the most devastating consequences of terrorism – we may end up living lives that are not worth living.

For Jennifer Edkins, "One of the most striking images of September 11 was that of people on the sidewalks in New York, their hands clasped over their mouths, transfixed in horror as they watched the impossible turning into the real in front of their eyes".[30] She argued that in this way, 9/11 had been "most characterized by silence":

> No cry was heard. Just the silent horror, as one cartoonist portrayed it, showing Edvard Munch's "The Scream" superimposed on the incredible landscape of the burning towers. Newspapers the following day printed nothing but pictures. And, in all the television coverage, time and time again, not a voiceover, but an image behind all the reports and discussions, as if to show, again and again, to anyone who hadn't seen it yet, that this was real.[31]

Edkins argues that the repetitive images of terrorism on 9/11 were so powerful – the timeless spectacle of the planes crashing into the Towers and the buildings collapsing – because they were witnessed by many millions of people, many in distant locations, through live, round-the-clock coverage. These images reminded witnesses in cities throughout the world that they have perhaps never been completely safe living and working there. More than this, 9/11 has shown city-dwellers that they are among the contemporary terrorists' target of choice. Witnesses in the city have rarely seen planes fall from the sky and buildings collapse. These possibilities have become the new post-9/11 coordinates of vulnerability and precariousness. It embodies a sudden awakening into a desert of the real where if New York can be so spectacularly targeted then why not London, Madrid, Sydney, Berlin, Paris or Melbourne? If people living and working in cities were the targets on 9/11 – and were again in Madrid on "3/11" and London on 7/7 – why wouldn't they be targets again? People can perhaps avoid injury by staying away from war-zones, but what can be done when the war zone – the strategic terrorist target – is a civilian city?

It was with these questions in mind that I conducted interviews with people living and working in the city of Melbourne, Australia in 2005. Through these interviews I was told stories. They were stories of living in a post-9/11 city whose inhabitants had been told that terrorism could occur at any time. Despite Melbourne never being the theater for a spectacular act of terrorism, I found people in this city deeply fearful of terrorism and the possibility of it disrupting their everyday lives. It is to these stories that I now turn.

Witnesses of Terrorism in the City

In my home city – Melbourne, Australia – there are many locations where a spectacular act of terrorism would spread tremendous devastation, fear and anxiety, produce terrifying images and, in turn, define Melbourne society for generations. An opportune image is presented to witnesses in Melbourne when they stand on the corner of Spencer Street and Collins Street – a major intersection in Melbourne's CBD. A turn to the left has the witness viewing the Rialto Towers; a huge skyscraper with an all glass façade. The Rialto was once the largest building in the Southern Hemisphere and it is home to a variety of corporate offices, restaurants and government workers.[32] A turn to the right has the witness facing the recently upgraded Southern Cross Station – a major public transport hub connecting the city with both regional and suburban locations.[33] This too is a building with a glass façade. Peering through the building, past the many train platforms, one can see the neon signs of Melbourne's second largest sporting stadium, *Etihad Stadium*.[34] The stadium has hosted many major events of social and cultural significance on a weekly basis, with attendances often in excess of 40,000 people. The stadium is home to several professional Australian Rules Football (AFL) teams, and also hosts cricket, major concerts (including AC/DC and the Red Hot Chilli Peppers) and national and international soccer and rugby fixtures. Across the road, is a plush new building (complete with a giant television screen facing the street and commuters) that is home to *The Age* newspaper – a major Melbourne daily. A few hundred meters to the left is the Herald Weekly Times office building, home of Australia's most read newspaper, the *Herald Sun*, and Australia's only daily national newspaper, *The Australian* (which are both News Ltd. Publications). Located in the inner suburbs of Melbourne a few short kilometers away are the offices of Melbourne's major television networks. In short, this one intersection in the Melbourne CBD is an ideal location for a terrorist spectacular, for the theater of terrorism.

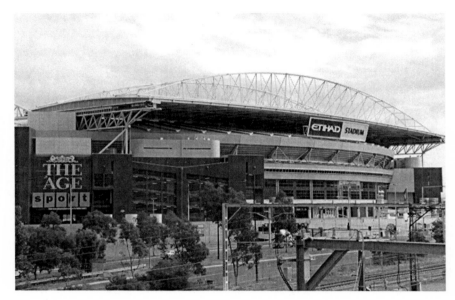

Etihad Stadium

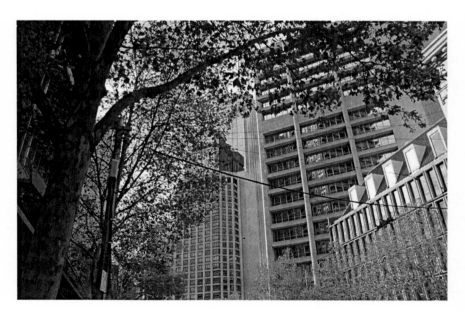

Rialto

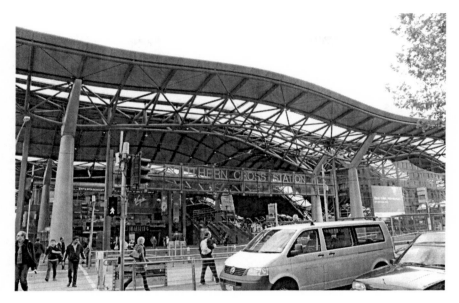

Southern Cross Station

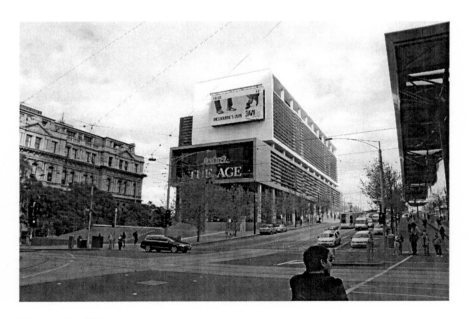

The Age Building

There would be many victims, incredible fear and terror, and, most importantly from the perspective of the fictional terrorists in this scenario, a global audience of witnesses via the mass media would be assured. In a way, Melbourne too is a traumascape of 9/11. I will give substance to this argument with the stories of Melbourne's witnesses of terrorism.

Since I conducted interviews with people living and working in Melbourne in 2005 I have been involved in a process of making sense of them, interpreting their meanings, and understanding the consequences of being a distant witness to terrorism. In many respects this was not difficult for me. I am a distant witness of terrorism, 9/11 in particular. 9/11 occurred on the evening of 11 September 2001 in South-Eastern Australia. In a surreal accident of fate, I was watching *West Wing* at the time. In an advertising break towards the end of the program the first reports of the attacks appeared on Australian television. At first, it was reported as an accident; a matter of an off course plane being unable to correct itself when traveling too close to a major city. It was not an implausible occurrence; most city-dwellers were perhaps aware of this possibility. It wasn't until *West Wing* concluded and round-the-clock coverage began in Australia that there was confirmation of something being wrong. It was not long before the second plane hit the other Tower; the South Tower. I felt so many emotions in that moment. I was horrified, disgusted, but also transfixed and – something that I am almost ashamed to admit – excited. Certainly this was not a happy excitement, nor a satisfying excitement. It was sickly, grotesque, a horrible and macabre theater of cruelty. But I could not look away. In fact, I was pretty sure others would be watching too.

Terrorism was not something entirely foreign to the average Australian at the time that 9/11 occurred. I will let the respondents in my research narrate for themselves later in this section. For me, terrorism tapped into a cultural and ethnic history. As an Irish Catholic – several generations of which had been born in Australia – I knew terrorism to be something that the IRA were accused of. When I had witnessed news reports in the 1980s of IRA terror, a terror which always seemed to be occurring in a far off land, I was reminded by my family, and my school teachers at a conservative, suburban Melbourne, Catholic primary school that violence was always regrettable, but sometimes necessary when used as a last option. It was in the years after 9/11 as I pursued my studies in terrorism and political violence, as well as in sociology and cultural studies, that I became more aware that terrorism had played a formative role in my life. I was never allowed to watch violent movies when I was young. Some of the blockbuster movies of my young life like *Predator, Nightmare on Elm St.* and *Robocop* were deemed by my family to be strictly off limits. Oddly, viewings of *The Omen* trilogy and the *Star Wars* trilogy were encouraged. The reasons why I was encouraged to watch *The Omen* movies is perhaps not difficult to understand. I am certain my family saw it as part of my religious education to see a simulation of the coming of ultimate evil. The Catholic and Christian themes in this film are unmistakable. The reasons I was encouraged to watch the *Star Wars* films, fairly violent movies when compared to other films I was not permitted to see, are perhaps less clear. For a long time I simply believed that my family did not want to rob me of experiencing a major cultural event. For many people, the *Star Wars* films were more than simply movies, they were also a cultural nexus; a representation of a zeitgeist of a particular time and place. But I now believe the reasons lie in the films' plot. At its core, *Star Wars* is the story of a legitimate insurgency, of guerilla warfare, and even terrorism. I was supposed to learn that sometimes violence is necessary against an unspeakable evil. Sometimes it is the government – the state – that is the illegitimate wielder of violence. The comparisons to the IRA's struggle should not need much explanation. It had been ingrained in me at a very young age that oft repeated saying; "*One person's terrorist is another person's freedom fighter*".

This was my 9/11. It is perhaps the 9/11 of someone who thinks about terrorism and popular culture a little too much, but since you are reading I can hardly make excuses for that. I spoke to other witnesses of 9/11 and terrorism who were living and working in Melbourne, Australia throughout 2005 in order to understand *their* 9/11s. In total I spoke with 105 people, 55 of whom I was able to interview at some length. I report on some of these interviews in this chapter. I cannot give a full account of all of the stories I collected in this research, but here I will highlight those accounts that most illuminate what it means to be a city dwelling witness of 9/11 and terrorism. Appropriately for my purposes in this book, I conducted these interviews under the methodological and ontological guidance of Donna Haraway's work on the "modest witness" and "situated knowledges". As I discussed in chapter one, these concepts are cornerstones in my understanding of witnessing and what I call a *sociology of we*. They have also been cornerstones for my thinking about terrorism. Through these theories, the interviews I have conducted, my PhD thesis and my first book I have come to view the witness as the central figure for understanding the meanings and consequences of terrorism.[35]

I have already used these interviews for other purposes. A full account of these interviews can be found in my book *Terrorism, the Worker and City: Simulations and Security in a Time of Terror*.[36] In that book I argued that contemporary terrorists have shown a particular penchant for targeting working people with their violence. I want to argue here that this penchant for targeting working people overlaps with a desire to localize many significant acts of terrorism in city spaces. In this way, the city has become the terrorists' visual playground; an ideal location in which to stage a terrorism spectacular.

The people I interviewed lived and worked in a major Australian city, a large, global metropolis in a world that is indefinitely described as *post-9/11*. They were witnesses of the 9/11 terrorist attacks. As was I. As were many millions of other people throughout the world. Many were witnesses in real-time, witnesses from a distance, and witnesses as part of a television audience. These interviews were conducted to explore the perceptions/subjective understandings of the meanings and consequences of terrorism in Melbourne, Australia's second most populous city. I have grappled with the information that I collected in these interviews over many months and years. These interviews provoked me to ask some fundamental questions about the meanings of terrorism, the meanings of witnessing, the meanings of television images, the meanings of spectacular violence, and how the threat of terrorism is at home in the contemporary city.

Toiling in the Desert of the Real

From the interviews a number of terrorism's meanings and consequences for city-dwelling witnesses emerged. Among these meanings and consequences were racism and discriminatory attitudes directed at people perceived to be Muslim, fear and anxieties associated with city working and city living, and a privileging of images of 9/11 in witnessing terrorism. There were also a number of idiosyncratic meanings and consequences but these three featured most prominently in the stories that these city-dwelling witnesses offered.

I conducted the first round of interviews on 21 February 2005 with people who worked in a retail organization located on an inner-city shopping strip in Melbourne's central business district (CBD). The first question I asked these witnesses was what terrorism meant to them. I chose this as my starting point in all the interviews I conducted because terrorism is a term and a concept with no widely agreed upon meaning. It would not have been reasonable to ask people questions about terrorism without first understanding what they understood as the meaning of "terrorism". As Patrick, a retail manager, described terrorism:

> Terrorism I think is, in my opinion, I believe it's [pause]. It's people [pause]. It's like [pause]. I can't really define it. I can give examples of it. I can't say, I can give you examples. Terrorism to me is like people, for example, like September 11, bombing the Twin Towers. Terrorism is suicide bombing. Terrorism is kidnapping people and executing them. All that kind of stuff.[37]

Responses like this were common. There was often some confusion at first, followed by a re-directing of the question I asked (*I can tell you what acts and events are terrorism even if I can't exactly tell you what terrorism is*), which was in turn followed, in almost every instance, with a reference to 9/11. As Paul, a retail employee, responded to the same question:

> Terrorism is [pause] someone who wants to affect the way that we live as a culture and live as a society [pause] someone who necessarily disagrees with my cultural views and wants to do their best to disrupt that ... my take on terror-

ism would be someone who fits certain stereotypes as well
… I think September 11 definitely brought it to the forefront
but other than that, it [terrorism] didn't mean anything to
us because, it is almost just because it wasn't used as often
[before September 11]. They spoke about it as much, but it
didn't mean as much to us.[38]

As I continued interviewing various people from differing age-
groups and workplaces, from different social classes and genders
it quickly became clear that 9/11 – even to these witnesses that had
witnessed the media reports of the Bali bombings in October 2003
that had killed 88 Australians – was the point of reference for understanding all "terrorism".

Indeed, of the 55 lengthy interviews that I conducted, all but
two described the 9/11 attacks as the most significant act of terrorism that they had witnessed. These two were senior managers at a
public transport organization that I interviewed shortly after the
London 7/7 attacks in 2005. Unsurprisingly, they believed that the
London 7/7 bombings that targeted people using the public transport network were the most significant attacks for them; the attacks
that had the most impact in their day-to-day lives as managers in
a public transport organization. Also significant in Paul's account
is his reference to "stereotypes" and the question of "who" is a
terrorist as a crucial feature of "what" terrorism is. This became a
significant outcome from this research. Most people I interviewed
admitted that they sometimes/often discriminated against people
that they perceived were Muslims. Some were regretful in recog-
nizing times when they acted in a discriminatory or racist way. Others were unapologetic, as Price, a defense employee, demonstrated:

The general gist is that it is Muslims [pause]. They are more
the terrorists [pause] the Muslims. *They* don't like the way
we have affected their lifestyle. *They* believe the things we
do in our general day would like, if *they* did that in their
country, it would cause some harm to themselves, it could
cause them to be killed. Whereas over here, it is just a normal everyday stuff. Everyone talks about it. *They* just think,
like, I wouldn't use jealous, but it seems like we are doing

something wrong, just living the way we do everyday. Just the things we do all the time.[39]

This view, which I would consider to be fairly intolerant and mostly uninformed, was decisively moderate when compared to some of the opinions of Muslims held by city-dwelling witnesses in Melbourne. Patrick was far less moderate in his perceptions of Muslims after 9/11:

> Terrorism and terrorists, especially when I worked at [Melbourne metropolitan shopping strip], I found it very difficult. When I think about terrorists and the terrorist threats I think about *the* certain race, I think about what's happening in Iraq, I think about people of that kind of race. As soon as I see one I think shit, you know. Especially if they are walking around [Melbourne shopping strip], I think to myself it is such a big complex and there are a lot of those people around there; it really wouldn't surprise me if something happened to that place. Like every time you hear a fire drill, an alarm, or you hear something happening, for example, like [pause] fire drills, the sirens, anything to do with that. You maybe think shit, something has happened and *they* are the first people you think about.[40]

Whilst Patrick in this part of the conversation does not mention Muslims or Islam, he makes several references to "the" race of people who he considers responsible for terrorism. But as our conversation continued it became clear who he considered "the" race to be.

> I certainly treated people differently. As soon as an Arabian, a Musso, as soon as a Muslim walked in, what I classified as a Mussi, I would genuinely try to stay away from them only because I didn't want to come into contact or have to deal with people like that. It sounds a bit racist but, just the mentality after September 11 and what you see on TV does make me have this kind of, I've given them a stereotype basically.[41]

Patrick has chosen the word "race" to describe people he believed adhere to Islam. This is, naturally, problematic since Islam is a religion that is observed by people of diverse racial backgrounds. But with this quote he qualifies his position. He considers "Arabians" and Muslims to be closely linked. The 2001 Australian census showed that the vast majority of Muslims (36%) are Australian born.[42] Of these, 30% reported a "Lebanese" ancestry. Many Australian Lebanese are Christian. Given this, it seems unlikely that Patrick might reliably be able to identify an Arabian Muslim. He seemed aware of this on some level and that his views were "a bit racist". For both Price and Patrick, identifying Muslims was closely related to identifying terrorism and terrorists.

The majority of respondents shared these views, although most were not proud of their beliefs. Some had an acute awareness that terrorism had changed who they were. Many seemed to know they were being racist and felt remorse for it. As Paul and I discussed:

> *Paul*: It's like, also another bad thing to say, a horrible thing to say, but you look at Aboriginals and I know for me, I class them as a certain type of people. Yet I know when I look at people who may look of an Islamic or Muslim faith and that sort of stuff, I class them as a type of people now.
>
> *Howie*: It's funny that they probably only have to look like they are Muslim.
>
> *Paul*: Exactly, and it may be that they are as Aussie as you or I but at the same time if they look a certain way, I judge them straight away. I don't consciously think about it. I don't remember any specific thing I have ever thought to myself but in my conscience I know it's there. Just thinking about it now. It comes to mind now. I know I must think it whenever I see them … my take on terror would be someone who fits a certain stereotype.[43]

Certainly, people experiencing fear and anxiety will sometimes deploy reductive, simplistic and stereotyping ways of thinking. The need to regain control of their fears, the need to blame and assign responsibility. These are the likely sources of their racism.

Fear and anxiety manifested in others ways for these witnesses. As Timothy, a legal clerk who works in a tall and prominent building in Melbourne's CBD, explained:

> It was just that after September 11, and then Madrid [a reference to the 3/11 attacks], that people who had to work, and had to get there with public transport, trains and stuff, suddenly felt different about things. You couldn't be sure anymore that, you know, something wouldn't happen. Because now we know they can.[44]

Fear and anxiety was often associated with mundane and routine daily activities for the witnesses I interviewed. Timothy in this instance described how fear and anxiety were now features of his commute to work in the post-9/11 world. Paul shared a story of how a routine fire alarm invoked the possibility of terrorism:

> *Paul*: A funny example is the other day on, I think I must have worked Wednesday. There was a fire alarm go off and everyone shit themselves and started walking out. And everyone was going, well what does that mean, what's going on. And everyone came up and said "I think it is a fire alarm, it's just a test". And others were like "nah, nah, that's not a fire alarm!" And now [pause].
>
> *Howie*: And did you hear the word terrorism used once or twice?
>
> *Paul*: Well, I didn't really, but you could just tell people were panicked like something was going on. It was like, *you know* … if anyone was going to try and make an impact. And that was the funny thing, you could just tell. Whenever there is a problem or some stuff like that people instantly think the worst.[45]

Whilst terrorism was not a pressing concern for Paul when he was working in the city, it was an everyday consideration when combined with mundane and banal routines. A fire alarm, in itself, is a common occurrence for anyone working in a building in Melbourne. Drills are a regular occurrence. For Paul, the threat of terrorism has given fire alarms new meanings. Paul believed that this was the purpose of terrorist attacks – to interrupt people's everyday lives. Terrorism was designed to create indefinite fear:

> I think it is more so just the fear that it could create. That we [terrorists] can inflict casualties anywhere, whenever we want. And you know, it could mean that geez! [They] create fear that, you know, what if I go here, what if they decide to do it there, what if I go here, you know. Will they do it there? I think it is more so the fear that it can create. It causes people to be worried about where they are going.[46]

For Timothy his fears were less related to "terrorism" than they were to "September 11":

> I don't know shit about terrorism. I know September 11. When I was watching the news, people immediately ringing up like radio stations, mosques and leaving abusive messages and threatening messages on the answering machines of the Muslim people. That's terrorism. If someone did that to me, rang me up and threatened me, obviously I'm going to feel scared. Being scared to me is terrorism. If you threaten someone and they feel intimidated or they feel unsafe, that's terrorism.[47]

Timothy's story highlights that 9/11 has had special consequences for people who live and work in cities. Many of the witnesses I interviewed were hesitant when talking about "terrorism" preferring instead to talk about what "9/11" meant to them. Time and time again in the conversations I had with witnesses I was told that 9/11 is something that was, in a way, more significant, more powerful, than "terrorism". Several of the quotes I have already shared showed that understanding terrorism was closely linked to 9/11 for these witnesses. As Paul described what it was like working in a city after 9/11:

[I held] a different view of the people that walked in after September 11. It's not something that I deliberately took upon myself to view people as. But it's just little messages that come through the media that it [terrorism] is possible.

Marcus, a consultant and small businessman who regularly found himself working for companies housed in tall and prominent buildings argued:

I used to work in the Rialto [a very tall and prominent building in Melbourne]. I was already a bit worried after September 11. One day our boss, or the building management, or something, got a call. It was the federal police saying that there is a concern about the Rialto for tomorrow and that you should tell your workers that they can work from home tomorrow. I was shit scared. We had just seen it happen [in New York].[48]

9/11 was a reference point, a watershed moment. It almost seems as though contemporary terrorism somehow began on that day for these witnesses. In symbolic terms, this may be close to the truth.

One of the more surprising responses in my research came from Allen, a partner in a prestigious Melbourne law firm housed in a tall and prominent building in the CBD. The following conversation took place between myself and Allen after I asked him whether terrorism affects his everyday life when working in the city:

Allen: No, not at all.

Howie: Really? [I look out the window at a view stretching out over the city and the bay] Because it would seem

Allen: Nope. Never.

Howie: Fair enough.

Allen: Well, I mean, of course I thought about it. How could I not?

Howie: Well, I …

Allen: I mean, look at it.

Howie: Yeah, no I agree.

Allen: It is harder to imagine though when you are in the building. I find it easier to picture when I am on the ground looking up.[49]

This is a quote that was of crucial importance to my research with city-dwelling witnesses of terrorism. This dialogue between Allen and I worked to foreground 9/11, tele-visual images of 9/11, and the precarious and vulnerable witness of terrorism in contemporary understandings of the meanings and consequences of terrorism. Allen's ability to best imagine the possibility of terrorism when he was standing outside of his building, looking up towards the floor where he works uniquely positions his feelings of terror within the traumascape of the city. Perhaps it also goes some way towards explaining why my colleagues and I paused to watch the plane pass by the Melbourne city skyline on the 7th anniversary of 9/11 (as I described in chapter one). The image was all-too familiar.

On and since 9/11 the most publicized and spectacular terrorism has occurred in the center of major cities and was traumatic for anyone who witnessed it. These targets were deeply symbolic. The Twin Towers, in particular, were powerful symbols of cosmopolitan and prosperous city-living. The attacks that destroyed them were so terrifying to distant witnesses in Melbourne because the Twin Towers reminded us that our city is full of tall and prominent buildings that house many thousands of city-dwelling witnesses. Skyscrapers in NYC; public transport in Madrid and London – these features can be found in any city throughout the world. For West and Orr contemporary acts of terrorism in city theaters have led to considerable "soul searching about security" amongst city-dwellers.[50] They argue that city spaces are, in a post-9/11 world, increasingly characterized by fearful, anxiety-ridden, angry and distrustful inhabitants. For these reasons city-dwellers have perhaps been far too receptive to new panoptic techniques. Even the value of torture routinely finds its way into the opinion columns of newspapers in major cities. In this way, cities will remain paradoxically "alarmingly powerful" (as a place of economic and labor hegemony, financial wheeling and dealing and a playground for the affluent) and "startlingly weak" (as a place of high crime and

a higher likelihood of becoming an actor in the theater of terrorism – the terrorists' visual playground).[51] It is this combination of
weakness and strength – of being a playground for the affluent and
the terrorist – that provokes violence. It also forces witnesses to ask
themselves some uncomfortable questions about the causes and
meanings of 9/11. *Are we targets of terrorism? Do terrorists have reason
to hate us? How are we to live as witnesses and victims of terrorism?*

Conclusion: Who Are the Targets of Terrorism?

> Go go speculator as you lead the charge of currency.
> Three trillion dollars a day you play with electronically.
> See that bleep on your screen? Do you realize what it fully
> means?
> Is this week's suffering in London, Skid Row or just Mexico?
> …
> Go! Go speculator. Trade up hard if the money's alright.[52]

> I'm your development corporation,
> spreading debt and disease across your nation.
> Breeding foreign debtors and a social decay,
> without a single election left to get in my way.
> What do you mean you want freedom too?
> Well there's not a damn thing that you can do.
> 'Cause I am rich and you are poor and all you control is
> petty national law …
> 51%, I own you.[53]

Whitaker argues that a crucial aspect of contemporary terrorism
is its random and arbitrary character.[54] He has described the 9/11
attacks as "out of the blue" and described the Madrid attacks on
3/11 as "unpredictable, random violence".[55] Yet terrorism is almost
never "random", "out of the blue" or even particularly "unpredictable". Indeed, terrorism is so dreaded and diabolical exactly because witnesses *can* reasonably imagine that terrorism might occur.
It is witnesses' abilities to anticipate cities as ideal theaters of terrorism that causes their fear and terror in response to global images of
violence.

On 9/11, the terrorists' violence was hardly "random". Indeed, attacking the economic nerve-centre and the military brain of one's enemy seems like an ideal way to strategically wage war – the US military's actions in Afghanistan and Iraq since 9/11 is perhaps compelling evidence of this. It is also possible that the plane that crashed in a field in Pennsylvania was on its way to the White-house, adding a third strategic target to the terrorists' crosshairs. In addition to these strategic considerations, New York City and Washington D.C. are among the most identifiable and well known cities on the planet. These cities are filled with city-dwellers going about their business, working and living in banal and routine ways. These cities were hardly random targets. Targeting these locations was sure to attract a global audience of witnesses. On 9/11, the tar-gets were carefully chosen, they were not drawn from a hat. The same holds true for the attacks in Madrid and London. These cities are global and recognizable, ideal theaters for terrorism. The unse-curable public transport networks were the focus of the violence. Terrorists were again successful in having a lot of people watching, not just a lot of people dead. I have argued elsewhere that on these days – 9/11, 3/11 and 7/7 – terrorists targeted working people to be the instrumental victims of their violent political agenda.[56] But it is just as clear that city-dwelling witnesses were the targets and the victims.

The witnesses that were interviewed were aware that they were the terrorists' targets of choice. They believed that terrorism – 9/11 in particular – had meanings and consequences for their lives in Melbourne; a city that has never been a theater for spectacular terrorism. These witnesses worked in this city, and formed a broad targeted group – city-dwelling witnesses, some of whom were working for global corporations. By targeting the Twin Towers in NYC, the economic nerve-center of the planet, the 9/11 terrorists sent a powerful message to corporate interests. Some have interpreted this message as *you are to blame*, at least partly, for the plight of underprivileged people throughout the world. Whilst news media outlets have tended to focus on the innocence of the victims in the Towers, others have pointed out that capitalism is viewed by some as an ultimate and pure evil, an evil that ensures that the rich become much richer and that the poor suffer and die.

This was the belief that underscored the quotes from the band *Insurge* that preface this conclusion. This is also among the claims of anti-globalization activists. The global financial crisis has, perhaps, strengthened their case – not only have some financial elites profited at the expense of the underprivileged, but also at the expense of the world economy and the middle-class elites that sustained it.[57] This was also at the heart of Ward Churchill's belief that the workers in the Twin Towers were legitimate targets of terrorism.[58] I explore this more fully in chapter four.

There is an irony in this argument. Osama bin Laden had built a billion dollar empire before 9/11 – he too was a beneficiary of globalized capitalism. Without the resources at his disposal, resources that provided access to communication and travel technologies, 9/11 would not have been possible. If the 9/11 hijackers were underprivileged and the oppressed, could they have carried out these attacks? Probably, but what form might their oppression have taken? They certainly enjoyed more privilege than billions of other people throughout the world who barely survive each day. It is at this point that we must ask *was the targeting of the economic heart of America a legitimate justification, or was it a rationalization and an excuse for terrorist violence?*

Turner argues that "Human beings are ontologically vulnerable and insecure, and their natural environment, doubtful".[59] To protect against some of the risks that people face, routine and everyday relationships and institutions are formed that come together to create what is often referred to as "society". People gravitate to these arrangements in the urban surroundings of the city. In the city, companionships and bonds are formed, rituals are entered and adhered to, common interests and pastimes are shared, various social and cultural institutions are forged. People go to work, students go to schools and universities. These institutions, places, spaces and locations in the city are themselves ontologically vulnerable and insecure like the people who dwell in them. The city is home to the wealthy and affluent, to industry and the worker. It is also the home of the corrupt, the criminal and the terrorist. The uncertainty that this creates does not undermine the prosperity of the city. It instead allows denizens to foster common bonds and share the risks and vulnerabilities characteristic of the city. This bonding leads to trust, empathy, and sympathy. Into the vulnerable city with its vulnerable denizens 9/11 was thrust as a violent event and an image. Contemporary terrorism was broadcast live into cityscapes. Whether near or far from terrorism's flashpoint, the possibility of terrorism is a routine and everyday part of life in the city.

The city is a *desert of the real*. It is also, therefore, home of the witness. Images of terror, the city and witnesses rely on each other for their existence. If violent images of 9/11 were not witnessed in distant cities then distant cities are not theaters. Yet without the city, and the targeting of cities on 9/11, there equally would be nothing spectacular for an audience to view. The spectacle of terrorism depends of the co-existence of witnesses, images of terrorism, and – in contemporary times – cities. 9/11 happened – it happened on 11 September 2001 in New York City, Washington DC and a field in Pennsylvania. The image, however, is not bound to this temporal and geographic logic. 9/11 was an atemporal event that can be understood in time and space in apparently unlimited coordinates of temporality and spatiality. It resides in the *desert of the real* of the contemporary city. It is also a place where powerful narratives of witnessing emerge.

3.

Celebrity Terrorism
Passion for the Real

The terrorists that CTU fights all day, every day, are both amply supplied and highly motivated. Some of their weapons are the same as our own. For the purpose of this manual, we highlight those weapons that terrorists use to instill fear in the populace. These are devices that either cause pandemonium and chaos or harm large numbers of innocent people – or both. (*Counterterrorism Unit Operations Manual*)[1]

The Fifth of November

Remember, remember the 5th of November.
Gunpowder, treason, plot.
I see no reason why gunpowder, treason
Should ever be forgot.[2]

From 26 to 29 November 2008, around a dozen coordinated attacks were carried out in Mumbai. When the smoke finally settled on the devastating events that had this city of more than 13 million people gripped in fear and terror, at least 170 people had been killed. During these attacks, that are sometimes referred to as "26/11", gunmen fired machine guns and threw grenades at various locations in "the heart" of Mumbai's commercial capital that included international hotels, a train station, a hospital, a movie theater and a Jewish center.[3] The goal of these terrorists was to elicit an exaggerated response from the Indian government, the global media and witnesses. These witnesses were sure to be many since "Almost within minutes, television screens showed harrowing scenes of pools of blood where people had died or been injured, hotels ablaze, Indian army snipers firing at distant targets, and CCTV images of the attackers".[4] Many of the images featured the attackers unmasked, seemingly proud to be on television. In this way the Mumbai terrorists were not unlike the parade of "normal" people that have appeared on so-called "reality" television programs. At times, the attackers are seemingly arching their backs and pausing so that their most terrifying angles can be captured as they hold machine guns and kill with impunity. At other times, gunmen can be seen walking casually, in mundane and banal poses whilst holding their guns as if to demonstrate perhaps the most terrifying aspect of these attacks – the terrorists were not out-of-control psychopaths; they were simply people, not necessarily unlike everyone else. Perhaps if we were to remove the guns, the bombs and the violence from these scenes in this Mumbai theater of terrorism, we might discover that terrorists act in ways not unlike celebrities – always seeking audiences, always trying to be captured as images in ways of their choosing, always trying to influence those who witness their antics.

These attacks were quickly described by Paul Cornish as representing an *"age of celebrity terrorism"*.[5] For a brief time, this term received some attention with Cornish's arguments circulating through newspapers throughout the world and the blogosphere. Certainly, terrorism has much in common with *cultures of celebrity*.[6] It is likely that it always has. Encoded in the word "celebrity" are ideas of witnessing and audiences, theaters, scenes and locations, actors, heroes and villains. As I have already argued in the previous chapters, terrorism involves all of these things, and always has. Like celebrity culture, if people are watching terrorism prevails. If few are watching terrorism fails. The London attacks of 7 July 2005 (7/7) provided a powerful example of this. These attacks have captured the imaginations of people living and working in the (Western) world's cities like few other attacks. London is a city of affluence and hegemony. When this city is attacked, witnesses take notice. On 23 July 2005 suicide terrorists bombed the Egyptian resort town of Sharm al-Sheikh killing 88 people;[7] a significantly larger number than the 56 that died in the 7/7 bombings. My intention is not to suggest that the 7/7 bombings were not significant – they remain devastating acts of terrorism of enormous destructive and symbolic power. But why do we remember the London bombings so much more clearly that the attacks in Egypt a few weeks later? Why were the attacks in Sharm al-Sheikh not commemorated with date coordinates – why are they not popularly known as the "7/23" bombings?

The short poem that prefaces this introduction is one example of how terrorism is *remembered*. This poem commemorates the night in 1605 when would-be terrorist Guy Fawkes and his Papist conspirators attempted an attack against Protestant parliamentarians in Britain at the Houses of Parliament.[8] To this day "Bonfire Nights" are held across the world to celebrate the 5th of November and the recent film *V for Vendetta* has glorified Guy Fawkes' planned attack.[9] The 5th of November perhaps should never – and will never – be forgot. How terrorism is "remembered" by global audiences of witnesses is particularly significant to those who seek to understand the motivations, goals and targets of contemporary terrorists. Of course, the 5th of November is not the only date that commemorates an infamous terrorist or terrorist attack. Symbolic date coordinates such as "9/11" (the spectacular live telecast of the attacks on New York and Washington DC and a field in Pennsylvania on 11 September 2001), "3/11" (the 11 March 2004 Madrid rail network bombings) and "7/7" (the 7 July 2005 bombings on the London public transport network) permeate everyday culture and ensure that the terrorism and terrorists from these dates are long remembered.

In this chapter, I intend to explain why some terrorism is remembered better than others. I suggest that the way we remember terrorism can, at least partly, be explained by exploring the powerful links between two seemingly disparate concepts; *celebrity* and *terrorism*. Terrorism has always, and will always be, designed to instill fear and terror in audiences of witnesses. If terrorism does not achieve this, then it is not terrorism at all. It should be called something else, probably "violence". But given the media zeitgeist of the 21st century it is perhaps unlikely that any significant act of violence would go unnoticed; and the news media are not the only producers of violent images. Writers and producers of television, film, and all manner of visual entertainment and screen cultures have long desired to tell tales of terror, violence and anxiety. These are also the industries from which celebrity cultures emerge. Walter Laqueur argued that "terrorism" has often been a attractive subject of popular culture.[10] But in a post-9/11 world we have witnessed a 9/11 popular, tele-visual and screen cultural frenzy as television and film creators have grappled for post-9/11 storylines for their productions – indeed, this frenzy helped inspire this book.

As such, this chapter progresses my arguments in this book substantially. It will bridge the gap between witnessing terrorism and 9/11's representation in popular, tele-visual and screen cultures. The idea of *celebrity terrorism* becomes a resource to this end. In one sense, this idea does little to advance our understandings of terrorism – terrorism, after all, has always been theater for living audiences of witnesses. However, celebrity terrorism brings contemporary terrorism into sharper focus and can work to make witnesses acutely aware that terrorists are attention seeking exhibitionists – just like the average Hollywood hunk or siren. With the popularity of television shows such as *24* (and a host of others, some of which I explore later in this book), we may also come to understand that terrorism is not only linked to celebrity, but that *terrorism is celebrity*. Terrorism fulfills what Žižek has described as our "passion for the real"; it is a passion that is also fulfilled by obsessions with celebrity cultures that take shape through celebrity gossip in the blogosphere, a place where reality and fiction become intertwined. It seems reasonable that we – as witnesses of 9/11 and of the post-9/11 world – might also follow celebrity terrorism to the blogosphere.

To explore these various dimensions of celebrity terrorism I have ordered this chapter in the following way; first, I map the new meanings that emerge when I bring together the seemingly disparate terms *celebrity* and *terrorism*. In doing so I outline what I consider to be the four fields for fusing these concepts – the terrorist as celebrity; locations for terrorism as celebrity; the celebrity as the target of terrorism; and the terrorism expert as celebrity. Following this, I share some examples of how the meanings of celebrity terrorism are depicted by witnesses of contemporary terrorism in what is sometimes called the "blogosphere".[11] I argue that since the blogosphere plays a significant role in the everydayness of celebrity culture, it should not be surprising that ferocious and often vitriolic debate surrounding the meanings of terrorism can also be found in weblogs. To this end I argue that the celebritization of terrorism is a natural and perhaps inevitable consequence of the intersections between contemporary terrorism, instantaneous and globalized internet and broadcast media and global audiences of witnesses. I conclude by arguing that television programs like 24 stand as confirmation that celebrity and terrorism are powerfully fused, and always have been. As Jack Bauer fights terrorism in real-time in the LA branch of the fictional CTU (Counterterrorism Unit), a real terror-war rages in the post-9/11 world. But any appeal to ideas of reality and fiction are problematic – 9/11 was a hyperreal event and fiction-like in its form and delivery. Our devout witnessing is symptomatic of our *passion for the real.*

Celebrity Terrorism

> To seriously cripple a society, terrorists often strike at its infrastructure. That is exactly what is accomplished with an electromagnetic pulse bomb or "E-bomb". The high-density electromagnetic field that results from the detonation of an E-bomb can wipe out all electronic devices within a substantial range ... weapons of this kind remain a very real and serious threat. (*Counterterrorism Unit Operations Manual*)[12]

My arguments in this chapter are based on the premise that some acts of terrorism are remembered better than others – some are captured by the news media's cameras even as they are occurring, some are recreated in feature films and television programs, while others are allowed to disappear and be forgotten. So whilst acts of terrorism like "9/11", "3/11" and "7/7" will perhaps never be forgotten, other attacks – such as those perpetrated by militant groups in occupied Iraq and Afghanistan, or perhaps those attacks carried out in non-Western locations – may be more quickly forgotten. I want to explain why this occurs by bringing together the seemingly disparate concepts of *celebrity* and *terrorism*.

The image and idea of *celebrity* plays a significant role in contemporary society and culture.[13] Graeme Turner has explored at length the meanings and consequences of celebrity and he is a pre-eminent scholar on celebrity culture.[14] One of Turner's most pressing concerns is the shift of celebrity to everyday, routine and banal realms. He describes this shift as "the demotic turn".[15] The demotic turn is "a means of referring to the increasing visibility of the "ordinary person" as they turn themselves into media content through celebrity culture, reality TV, DIY websites, talk radio", and it represents "celebrity's colonization of the expectations of everyday life in contemporary western societies".[16] Moreover, Turner argues that the demotic turn might be elsewhere deployed to understand other fields of "relations between media and culture".[17]

It is at these points of "relations" between media and culture that I locate this discussion of celebrity terrorism. As Cornish argues, terrorists seeking celebrity "indulge in terrorism simply because they can, while their audience concocts a rationale on their behalf".[18] The goals of the celebrity terrorist are notoriety, fame and the production of terrifying and powerful images that have meanings and consequences far beyond the "flashpoint" of terrorist violence.[19] They are "ordinary" in a way and their spectacular violence makes them visible. It is through terrorism that they are witnessed. For Cornish, "the character of modern terrorism" is powerfully shaped by its image producing power and its spectacular consequences.[20] When terrorists are able to launch acts of terrorism capable of producing spectacular and violent images that attract audiences of witnesses, they give their violence every chance of being remembered. As I identified in chapter one, the desire to create powerful images has long been a crucial goal for terrorists. According to Jenkins terrorists seek to have a lot of people watching, not just a lot of people dead.[21] It has been suggested that the result of this is an audience of witnesses that perceive terrorism as posing a danger far greater than any damage that terrorists could realistically cause.[22] For would-be terrorists, being seen is perhaps more important than achieving some sort of concession from a government or military authority. Colen, writing in the conservative online magazine *The Brussels Journal*, disparagingly describes the terrorists' desire to be seen as "Paris Hilton Terrorism" – it is a type of terrorism that privileges visibility over achievement or success.[23] Or, more precisely, where *visibility is the achievement or success.* It may be that in the world of the spectacle terrorist and celebrities like Paris Hilton, any publicity is good publicity. In Colen's cynical analysis of the meaning of celebrity terrorism she argues that terrorists "crave ... what Paris Hilton and Madonna crave for when they have sex in public. What they long for ... [is] an obsessive audience"; an audience of witnesses that will turn everyday terrorists into media celebrities.[24]

The Terrorist as Celebrity

Long before 9/11, Ben Perrin noted something that many terror-ism studies scholars were mostly ignoring – a "fundamentalist's banker", "the world's pre-eminent financier of anti-American ter-rorism", and a "bashful superstar" was receiving increased fame and notoriety amongst radicalized and revolutionary communities throughout the world.[25] The man that Perrin was referring to when he wrote his short opinion piece in 1998 was Osama bin Laden. Following the attacks that targeted two US embassies in Northern Africa in 1998 and the retaliation attacks that destroyed a pharma-ceutical company and devastated the population of the Sudan, bin Laden became "a hero in life and would be a martyr in death to his brothers and sisters".[26]

> His plight has been elevated. Funds will be easier to raise, new recruits more expedient to muster and international contacts more diverse. There is no doubt that Bin Ladin was involved in dubious activities before last month's embassy bombings, but now he has been singled out and thus made a celebrity in his own way.[27]

In a strange twist the date of Perrin's article is 11 September 1998. The terror attacks in North Africa and the path to 9/11 was forged through the celebritization of Osama bin Laden. He became some-one who could not simply be killed since his death may have led to him being lionized – he had the potential to become the terror-ist version of Kurt Cobain or Jeff Buckley. In short, his increasing fame needed to be contained. Tragically, his fame became a vessel through which 9/11 became possible.

Nacos frames terrorism as "celebrity" when it receives "saturation coverage" making "the perpetrators of mass-mediated political violence excellent candidates for celebrity status".[28] Certainly, it seems uncontroversial to suggest that media reporting of terrorism may be a site for the construction of celebrity terrorism. This was, according to Nacos, best exemplified by the media reporting in the aftermath of the Oklahoma City bombing and, in particular, the reporting leading up to the perpetrator's – Timothy McVeigh's – execution. He became, in many respects, "just like O.J. Simpson or Princess Diana".[29] She argues that the media turned Timothy McVeigh into a celebrity, spectacularized his violence and provided him with a larger audience of tele-visual witnesses.[30] Osama bin Laden has similarly received this celebrity treatment.[31] Nacos notes that "bin Laden didn't have to say or write anything to dominate the news" in the aftermath of 9/11.[32] Undoubtedly, when the news media reports on terrorism it can be difficult for witnesses to look away.

A recent event in Australia's theater in the "War on Terror" represents an illustrative case of an accused "terrorist" quickly becoming a celebrity. Dr Mohammed Haneef became an instant celebrity in 2007 when the Queensland-based, Indian-born doctor was detained for ill-defined and mysterious terrorism offences. Dr Haneef was celebritized as a terrorist with little critical reflection or sound intelligence and policing analysis. The difference between Haneef and other terror celebrities such as McVeigh and bin Laden is that Mohammed Haneef had absolutely no connection to terrorism, played no role in any act or planned act of terrorism, and was – unsurprisingly – not a terrorist. When the media produces a terrorist as a celebrity however, innocence or guilt plays little role. Amongst the comical analysis in the media of terror threats and dangers that the detaining of Haneef sparked, anything constituting a "fact" was difficult to come by.[33] What we know is that on 30 June 2007 an amateurish attempted terrorist attack took place at Glasgow Airport. On 2 July 2007 a so-called "link" was determined between the attempted attack and Mohammed Haneef and he was subsequently arrested and detained without charge under Australia's controversial post-9/11 terror laws. There was a frenzied journalistic response. Button, writing in the Melbourne daily left-liberal newspaper, *The Age*, described how British police were "desperately trying to establish a common denominator" between the failed Glasgow attack and Dr Haneef.[34] Crawford and Hudson writing in Australia's most popular tabloid newspaper, the conservative *Herald Sun*, reported that people were ringing hospital switchboards to ensure that family and friends were not being treated by terrorists.[35] Greg Pemberton writing in the conservative *The Australian*, Australia's only national daily newspaper, noted that policing authorities had "not yet made a link" between Haneef and the attempted attacks in Glasgow, but he then bizarrely concluded:

> But the timing of events, the acknowledged British source of advice and the fact one of the men arrested, Mohammed Haneef, was a registrar at Gold Coast Hospital in Southport, so a doctor, who had trained in India before coming to Australia from Northern England, suggest a direct connection.[36]

Did it suggest a direct connection? Hardly. Muslims can at least be grateful that such circumstantial evidence that would place perhaps hundreds of Australian doctors in a position of "direct connection" with terrorism would not stand-up to legal scrutiny. Analysis such as this, book-ended with claims that "We may have dodged a bullet", worked to celebritize Dr Mohammed Haneef as a terrorist. Despite later reports of possible police bungles in handling the case, secret plots to make the charges stick, and Haneef's total exoneration of any wrongdoing, the celebritization of Dr Haneef as a terrorist had already occurred.[37]

These accounts of celebrity terrorists – embodied in the figures of Timothy McVeigh, Osama bin Laden and Dr Mohammed Haneef – show that the media will quickly thrust real terrorists and short-term terrorist suspects into the headlines. Terrorism, like sex, sells. The media are motivated by a desire for profit, market share and notoriety to sensationalize even the most mundane terrorist events. In the process, terrorists are handed an easy victory and earn notoriety and celebrity-status. Yet the celebritization of the terrorist – which has been the focus for all accounts of celebrity terrorism to date – is only part of the story. There are many other fields in which terrorism is celebritized. Among these are some familiar, albeit inanimate, post-9/11 celebrities.

Locations for Terrorism as Celebrity

How far should my analysis of celebrity terrorism extend? Should it extend to places and objects? Certainly New York City and the Twin Towers were already among the most well known images of a Western city before 9/11, but could it not also be argued that the 9/11 terrorist attacks made NYC and the Twin Towers among the most *seen and witnessed* cities and locations in human history?

Through 9/11, the Twin Towers and NYC have attained a renewed *celebrity* status. In a post-9/11 world, NYC and the Twin Towers share something in common with Paris Hilton, Brad Pitt and Britney Spears – people want to see them, people want to know about them, and when their images appear on television and in other media spaces it is difficult for witnesses to look away. It is in this context that post-9/11 NYC and the Twin Towers are uncredited stars of some situation comedies that were/are symbolically set in NYC. In post-9/11 episodes of *Friends* and *Sex and the City* the Twin Towers were purged from all the wide-angle shots of NYC that were used to join scenes and accompany the opening credits (I explore this in detail in chapter four). More recently *How I Met Your Mother* has continued this trend of forgetting 9/11. The absence of the Twin Towers from pop cultural representations of New York is distracting, and perhaps an indication of some deeper and horrific trauma of being terrorism's living witnesses. I originally viewed *How I Met Your Mother* as evidence of an American and global culture that was eager to forget, to disavow 9/11 in order to recover from its consequences. However, Carter Bays, one of the program's creators, explained in an interview that his show and its narrative technique of story-telling the present from an imaginary future is designed to be a tribute to post-9/11 NYC:

> It's just that, almost immediately after 9/11, it felt like there was this sense of nostalgia for a time that wasn't too long ago because all of a sudden the world was different. There was this sense of looking at these days right now as the future good old days because you never know what's going to happen. It felt nice to think, as scary as the world is now, about a version of ourselves telling this story 30 years from now … It means the world didn't blow up.[38]

How I Met Your Mother stands as a metaphor for a better post-9/11 today – a today that will be retold and reanimated at some later point as a wonderful time to be alive, fall in love, and recover from the tragedy and trauma that had accompanied the beginning of the 21st century.

The Celebrity as the Target of Terrorism

If we are entering an age of celebrity terrorism then the next logical development may be terrorists targeting celebrities to be the victims of their symbolic violence. This type of celebrity terrorism was witnessed in early 2009 when the Sri Lankan cricket team was attacked in the Pakistani city of Lahore. Six policemen who were escorting the Sri Lankan team bus and the bus driver were killed. Seven cricketers, including experienced international players Kumar Sangakkara and Chaminda Vaas (household names in the cricketing world), sustained serious gunshot wounds.[39] It was reported that ten to twelve gunmen ambushed the Sri Lankan cricket team on its way to a Test match at Gaddafi Stadium. Soon after the attack commenced (a matter of minutes), images were being beamed across the globe. Global media audiences witnessed the Pakistani security forces surrounding the Sri Lankan team bus to reach survivors but they failed to capture any of the terrorists. But viewing audiences were left in little doubt that sporting personalities were ideal targets for spectacular acts of terrorism.[40]

In 2009 the American singer Heather Schmid – a performer who is particularly popular in China and Pakistan – had reportedly become a target of al-Qaeda because of her support for the Pakistani government and her friendship with President Musharraf.[41] As she explains:

> I started to get disturbing phone calls and Facebook requests, my Web site was being hacked in a very slow, clever way. Things like my family photos were being taken and my tour schedule was changed. My webmaster tracked it back to Pakistan … my friend was shocked to find an extremist video on YouTube where myself, Condoleezza Rice and President Bush are the Americans in the video considered as "Anti-Islamist".[42]

Former Beatle Paul McCartney has similarly attracted the ire of pro-Palestinian groups by performing in Israel as part of the nation's 60th anniversary celebrations. A Syrian Sheik, Omar Bakri Mohammed, has suggested that McCartney is "the enemy of every Muslim" because his performance in Israel offered support to an anniversary that celebrates the "atrocities of the occupiers".[43]

This represents an alarming – but also logical – shift in the tactics of terrorists. Perhaps terrorists are no longer satisfied with perpetrating spectacular *violence* when a more spectacular *target* will be a far more effective way of attracting attention, gaining celebrity status and spreading terror. Just as al-Qaeda terrorists know that 3000 dead Americans in New York City are worth far more than 3000 dead American soldiers in the Iraqi and Afghan deserts, the terrorist who targets celebrities knows that a dead celebrity may send a more powerful message than a dead non-celebrity. Indeed, paparazzi photographers would perhaps already be pointing cameras at celebrities at the moments they were targeted by terrorists. In this way celebrity terrorism will tell witnesses more about how terrorism is remembered than it will about the terrorists' political grievances.

Terror Academicus: The Terrorism Expert as Celebrity

It has often been claimed that everything changed on 9/11. It seems clear that the academic world was not immune to the power of 9/11 to generate change. Amongst the sometimes strange consequences of 9/11 rests the rise of the *terrorism academic*. Before 9/11 there was a dedicated group of scholars that investigated the meanings and consequences of terrorism and these scholars have, rightly, remained household names in the contemporary terrorism studies canon. However, 9/11 became the launching pad for an avalanche of terror scholarship and career academics – being 21 years old when 9/11 occurred, I am undoubtedly part of this group that is sometimes disparagingly referred to as the "new-school" of terrorism studies. This new-school is sometimes considered to be a little idealistic and often naïve. As someone who was trained in more classical terrorism studies, I find it hard to disagree. Regardless of one's perspective on the state of terrorism studies in academia, there is little doubt that there has never been so many opinions and arguments about the meanings and consequences of terrorism and never have so many people studied *terrorism*. This rise in *terror academicus* was accompanied by a media frenzy where journalists were eager to break stories on subjects that have anything to do with terrorism. Some of these new-school academics have become terror celebrities in their own right, some deservedly, others problematically.

In a study conducted by David Miller and Tom Mills ranking the most frequently interviewed terrorism academics in English language media throughout the world, the authors argue that "Terrorism experts are ubiquitous in mainstream media coverage of political violence".[44] They argue that terrorism academia is a problematic and ideologically driven field: "We see terrorism knowledge not as some ideologically neutral expertise on a natural phenomenon, but as being created to reflect the priorities and values of certain social interests".[45] Miller and Mills also track the unsurprising corresponding rise in the reporting of terrorism post-9/11. Prior to 9/11, terrorism experts are said to have occupied an "invisible college" of dedicated scholars who crossed over with many other fields of political science and social science inquiry including counterinsurgency studies, Cold War studies, international relations, politics, anthropology, sociology and a host of other sub-disciplines. In a post-9/11 world terrorism academics are an everyday feature of most Western universities. This would all be unproblematic if traditional terrorism scholars were as well represented in Miller and Mills' rankings as the new-school terrorism scholars are. But this is not the case. The reasons for this, in many instances, is not entirely clear, but it seems likely that terrorism scholars that reach out to journalists and offer sensational analysis will be more likely to receive air-time. Sadly, the terrorism academic's command of special expertise in the field of terrorism studies will sometimes have little to do with who appears in the media. Having often appeared in the media discussing terrorism I have learnt that controversial opinions, a failure to provide pithy sound bites, and an unwillingness to respond to simplifications will often lead to my opinions being omitted from the story. Offering expert opinions to the media on terrorism is a challenging experience. My most common experience with journalists has involved receiving a call during which I am asked to provide my opinion on a particular issue relating to terrorism. I respond explaining my expertise and what I would be comfortable commenting on. This is often the end of the road. Unless I am prepared to engage in some speculative guess-work about what terrorists were thinking as they carried out an attack or unless I am willing to "make the call" and state for the record who carried out the attack and why, I will, most likely, receive no air-time. Unfortunately there are throngs of academics ready to respond with speculative commentary and sensationalistic opinions and willing to engage in the guess-work that journalists seem to require.[46]

This phenomenon has received some attention. Kevin Toolis, writing for the *New Statesman*, argued in 2004 that whilst the "study of terrorism is booming" many of the terrorism experts "represent an ideology that has its roots in the cold war and in Israeli conservatism".[47] Toolis's arguments have some merit but he is deeply misguided in identifying targets for ridicule. He goes on to describe some of the most respected terror academics of the twentieth century as post-9/11 "guns for hire".[48] Petra Bartosiewicz argues that the emergence of the post-9/11 terror academic has "significantly affect[ed] the way the "war on terror" is framed, investigated and prosecuted".[49] Blogger "Dick Destiny" frames this phenomenon as the "Celebrity Terrorism Expert".[50] He argues that they are "Always there to connect the dots on television or in news articles and opinions, the celebrity terror expert has all the right answers. It's a convenient gig".[51] Dick Destiny believes that some terrorism experts are peddlers of information that will get their faces on television: "whatever message needs a push, the celebrity terrorism expert is there to provide it".[52]

These accounts of celebrity terrorism are intended as a starting point; little more than a map of how celebrity and terrorism might be understood in the same space. These four dimensions of celebrity terrorism – the terrorist as celebrity; locations for terrorism as celebrity; the celebrity as the target of terrorism; and the terrorism expert as celebrity – stand as signposts for understanding some of the ways that terrorism and celebrity cultures intersect to create a greater audience of witnesses. It is reasonable to believe that the acts of terror I referred to in previous sections would have had a less significant impact if they had not been *celebritized*. A machine gun attack in Pakistan attracts some attention, when the Sri Lankan cricket team is the target it attracts much more. When an act of terror occurs it attracts some attention. When that act of terror is linked, no matter how spuriously, to al-Qaeda or one of their amorphous so-called regional affiliates, it attracts more. Such is celebrity terrorism, where the quest to be remembered has lead to some spectacular images of violence.

Remember, Remember: Witnesses of Terrorism in the Blogosphere

> Each day, terrorists plot to wreak wanton violence upon the citizens of this nation. At times, it may be necessary for CTU agents to use excessive force – i.e., torture – to ensure the rapid conclusion of a mission. New agents sometimes find it difficult to comprehend or condone some of the methods the agency uses to carry out interrogations. Torture is distasteful and rightfully deplored by all good citizens of the world. But the judicious use, or the threat, of torture can be an effective tool to extract information. (*Counterterrorism Unit Operations Manual*)[53]

In my attempts to locate those who have also fused terrorism with celebrity by conducting literature searches of the usual kind (library databases and book searches, online mining, Google and Google Scholar searches, sifting through newspapers from around the world on online databases and microfiche) I discovered that, not unlike celebrity cultures more generally, celebrity terrorism was being grappled with in the blogosphere. In this section, I explore the responses of some of these bloggers. They are witnesses of terrorism of a different kind to the witnesses featured in the previous chapter. It is not my intention to conduct a rigorous survey of the blogosphere. Rather, I want to explore these bloggers accounts as *located witnesses*; witnesses that offer accounts of what they witnessed in virtual, online spaces. Naturally, I am not the first to explore the blogosphere in an attempt to illuminate the meanings and consequences of social and cultural worlds and I do not consider methodological purity in blog research to be what is at stake in this chapter.[54] Rather, my exploration of the blogosphere was motivated by there being something about the word "terrorism" that, at times, sends the blogosphere into frenzied and vitriolic debates. My motivation was also to track witnesses of terrorism through this often ignored field in screen and visual cultures.

So far in this chapter I have mapped the contours of celebrity terrorism. In some respects, celebrity terrorism is little more than a re-articulation of long held beliefs in the study of terrorism and the media – terrorists seek media attention; the media aids the spread and consequences of terror; terrorism is theater; the media is the *oxygen* of terrorism.[55] Terrorism, as I have already argued in this book, is theater for living audiences of witnesses, and I have shown in chapter one that this is not new. But celebrity terrorism represents more than this. Celebrity terrorism highlights that "terror" involves more than actors and television cameras. It involves witnesses. We must follow these witnesses to the places where they watch, where they bear witness. I have followed celebrity terrorism into the blogosphere.

Throughout the world internet users crowd the blogosphere to gossip about the latest antics of Hollywood, sporting, political and all manner of random and temporary celebrities. Unsurprisingly, celebrity gossip in the blogosphere has been easily extended into gossip about terrorism. Piers Morgan, editor of the British celebrity-obsessed tabloid, the *Mirror*, argued in October 2001:

> [P]erhaps for the first time in 30 years, people in this country [Great Britain] are rejecting the Big Brother-style trivia they so adored five weeks ago and realizing there really are more important things in the world ... There is a sudden and prolonged hunger for serious news and information.[56]

But this search for "serious news and information" did not lead internet gossip junkies to abandon their blogs – indeed, they re-animated the blogosphere with post-9/11 banter. This is, I suggest, a powerful demonstration of Turner's "demotic turn" at work. The blogosphere has become a location where everyday witnesses of terrorism can become terrorism experts and quasi-celebrities through the public airing of their opinions. No longer is the media dominated solely by those not-so-select and swelling crew of terrorism studies "experts" who comment on terrorism and security, often with dubious speculation. In witnessing the war on terror, dubious speculation has become everybody's right. In this way, celebrity terrorism takes the "demotic turn" and this specific type of celebrity reaches the realms of the everyday through sometimes furious, sometimes measured, debates and articulations in the blogosphere.

In the aftermath of the Mumbai "celebrity" terror attacks, the blogosphere temporarily filled with such terror banter. Some of these blogs were positioned as responses to Cornish's arguments about celebrity terrorism. As "Irco" writes in a blog hosted by *digg.com*:

> we've already come to a point where people would pretty much do anything to appear on a tv show (see reality shows). Even though the thought of "celebrity terrorism" to that scale hadn't crossed my mind until now, I still think it is highly possible that there would be people out there just craving for the attention ... it's pretty ***** up.[57]

A disdain for people who would "do anything to appear on tv" was, according to Turner, a typical response after 9/11. Turner argues that as a consequence of the "real" that images of 9/11 delivered to witnesses, a distaste for tabloidization and vain attention-seekers led to a significant decline in demand for celebrity themed magazines and celebrity based talk-shows, and reality-television programs scheduled for the US winter ratings seasons were "drastically culled".[58] Television programs featuring humiliation and fear – programs like *Fear Factor* – were suddenly unpalatable to media audiences. It is interesting to note that during the months following 9/11, the television program *Friends* experienced renewed popularity (a full account of this can be found in chapter four). In short, post-9/11 television audiences demanded more from networks than sloppy 15 minutes of faming and degrading reality slap-togethers – 9/11 had perhaps stocked witnesses with enough humiliation and reality for the time being. Or perhaps media audiences were tired of terror and human suffering as entertainment since this was also the form of terrorists' propaganda by the deed.

This propaganda was a crucial aspect of Cornish's belief that the Mumbai attacks represented celebritized terrorism. He suggests that:

> In a novel twist, the Mumbai terrorists might have embarked on propaganda of the deed without the propaganda in the confident expectation that the rationalization for the attack – the narrative – would be provided by politicians, the media and terrorism analysts.[59]

Cornish added that the Mumbai attacks were designed to inspire other would-be terrorists to similarly carry out their violent desires (in arguing so, he seemingly misses the point that *this* would be the propaganda's target and content, with the violence as the deed). The Mumbai terrorists had undoubtedly hoped their violence would incite "the world's D-list malcontents" to violently pursue their own radical desires for notoriety and fame without needing to be articulate, wealthy or particularly educated (famous for being famous).[60] In this way, the celebrity terrorists' fame would be something closely akin to the fame experienced by reality television celebrities – temporary but powerful. However, as the blogger "domiciliphile", also hosted at *digg.com*, argues:

> I think what was different in the Mumbai attacks is being misinterpreted by the author [Cornish], perhaps even propagating a problem of interpretation through a myopic Western lens. In fact, I think we have to be careful, because I believe "Celebrity terrorism" is just a failed attempt at sandwiching two separate and distinct, revenue-generating buzz words together, and ultimately, terrorists will only be as "celebrity" as we make them.[61]

Celebrity terrorism may indeed be a "revenue-generating buzz word", but it is also a powerful way of framing the meanings and consequences of contemporary terrorism, its image producing power, and the ways that terrorism is remembered and witnessed. The term suggests that as long as there are people willing to pay attention, watch and witness when terrorism occurs, terrorism, terrorists and their targets will receive a celebrity's share of attention.

This occurs whether terrorists are "real" or "imagined", produced through counterterrorism policing errors, or produced by "expert" commentary and journalistic spin. All of these factors contributed to the celebritization of Dr Haneef and of so-called Somali terrorists in Australia as I will explore later in this section. Hot on the heels of counterterrorism police, terrorism experts and the media are blogger-witnesses. Or, perhaps blogger-witnesses do not trail at all – many might prefer the bloggers and rely on them to provide more grassroots, perhaps more real and grounded, commentary.

I have been from time to time particularly interested in those more-or-less anonymous blogs that appear at the end of newspaper articles in some major tabloidized publications. One such publication in Australia is News Corporation's *Herald Sun*. The *Herald Sun* has a flair for sensationalizing major and mundane events alike. I read many online newspapers from many cities throughout the world and I am sad to say that this Melbourne daily sits well amongst the most conservative and most-sensationalistic in mainstream journalism. Since it is read by nearly 1.5 million people each day, it is also influential.[62] Among the features that this newspaper's online version offers is a real-time blog that accompanies the most controversial articles (which, through some journalistic spin, is most articles). On 4 August 2009 a sensationalized terror scare hit the pages of the *Herald Sun*. The headline read: "Four Arrests in Terror Swoop".[63]

The article briefly explains that four alleged terrorists of "Somali and Lebanese descent" had been arrested for planning a machine gun attack against an Australian army barracks in Sydney (as my colleagues have pointed out to me, a planned attack that was doomed to fail given that the facility that was the target is reportedly home to crack counterterrorism forces). This attack was limited in scope and since the planned target was a military facility, the notion that this was "terrorism" is highly problematic. Yet, as the blog posts following this article show, this planned attack was successful in generating a ferocious and vitriolic response from *Herald Sun* readers. It was a response forged by fear and terror, and one filled with racist language and bigotry. The blog responses form a powerful case of how easy it is to overreact in the face of terror, how audiences of witnesses react in the immediate aftermath of terror reporting, and how internet screen cultures are locations in which terrorism can be understood and witnessed.

With scant details at hand, the bloggers unleashed a tirade directed at immigrants and foreigners, the accused, other imagined would-be terrorists and their so-called sympathizers, and anyone who disputes the supposed dangers and risks posed by international terrorism. As the first commenter, "Andy", in the post-article blog argued with simplicity and symbolic xenophobia: "Islam, the religion of peace!!!!!!!!!!!!!!!!".[64] The second commenter, "Marty of ringwood" shared similar emotions:

> *We* allow these people to come into Australia as refugees ... desperately running away from terror in their countries. Then they enjoy the peace and freedom *we* have here. But the ungrateful sods ... have the audacity to start terror cells and have plans to attack army bases in Australia ... I think *we* should rescind their Citizenship rights and send them back to where they came from ... They become Australians and then feel safe to carry out their dastardly deeds against the very people who have given them sanctuary.[65]

I have italicized "we" when it appears in this post to emphasize the way the author has used the word in his discussion of terrorism. As I indicated in chapter one, the word "we" is often used in discussing terrorism and in the desperate attempts to classify enemies and allies during terror scares. It was reported widely soon after the attacks that the accused attackers were "Australian citizens".[66] Indeed to send some of them "home" would mean sending them to suburban Melbourne. Despite this their Lebanese-ness and Somali-ness immediately excluded them from the category of "we". As blogger "AJ of Boronia" sarcastically wrote, "Welcome to the future of Melbourne. Multiculturalism is thriving here".

The vast majority of the blog contributions in the immediate aftermath of this story were based on a discourse of the need for immigration restrictions, cracking down on "Muslims" and the "sending home" of terror suspects. Yet, a few bloggers reminded their fellow bloggers that this story may amount to no substantial threat at all. As "Asianplumb of Melbourne" wrote: "Surveillance of an army base might just mean google earth? Plotting could mean having a conversation of hypotheticals? Let's hope the federalies have more than just maybes and this isn't another Haneef style embarrassment?". Similarly, "Liz of Melbourne" writes

> Just as pathetic as these terrorists … are the white terrorists writing here. So far I've read "inspired by" and "one of them", I haven't heard anything about weapons or explosives being found. Basically the Anglo-Saxon race will use anything they can get their hands on to utilize for their "accepted" racism. *We have a crapload of Muslims and 99% are like the rest of us.* Basically most of you [other bloggers] loved this opportunity to be a temporary public racist … that's all. Remember Dr. Haneef … you were saying the exact same thing.[67]

Overwhelmingly, these sentiments were the minority view. "Keith of Melbourne" was particularly vitriolic:

> Time for Australia to suspend ALL Islamic immigration. At least until this so-called peaceful religious group show evidence globally of no longer planning attacks against innocent civilians in the name of their god? Just how many billions of dollars have been spent (wasted) worldwide since the events in New York, Bali, UK, and Jakarta perpetrated by this group of religious fanatics? Obviously only a small percentage of Muslims are responsible for these acts, but until we have a better method of identifying and weeding out the culprits, AND perhaps the self policing by the peaceful Muslims, I would prefer that no more are admitted to Australia.[68]

I could go on and on with quotes like this. When I printed the post article blog some two hours after the blog began, there had been 478 comments, almost all expressing some version of the "send them home", anti-Muslim, anti-immigration agenda.

At the time of writing in March 2010, there had been few updates on the status of the detained "Lebanese" and "Somali" terror suspects. However, there has been a sudden and dramatic escalation in fears of terrorists emerging from Africa. Hastily, the group that the arrested terror suspects were allegedly inspired by, al-Shabab, was added to lists of banned terrorist organizations (despite this group being best known for fighting over territory, not religious ideal-ism). Adding fuel to the fire was a new government white paper on terrorism, released in February 2010, warning that terrorism in Australia will likely emerge from "within".[69] It would be fair to say, however, that the threat posed by these suspected terrorists who were Australian-citizens of African and Lebanese origin was mini-mal. But this does little to soften the blow for Australia's Muslims and immigrant communities – the damage had been done. Austra-lians were suddenly aware of a new category of terrorist celebrities – Somalis and other Africans. They have taken their place alongside the traditional suspected terrorist category "Muslim". They are the new terror celebrities and any Somali or African is, for some, a po-tential terrorist – at least until Australians are distracted by another group that can be celebritized.

In the film *Starship Troopers* audiences witness a war being waged by the human race against alien bugs from space.[71] In one of the film's most memorable scenes we see children and a woman on Earth jumping on the sidewalk in some wealthy suburban lo-cale shrieking hysterically as they squash garden variety bugs, as though it somehow helped the war effort against the giant bugs in space. One of the film's catch-cries is "The only good bug is a dead bug!".

This story is a metaphor for how some react to witnessing ter-rorism (or the threat of terrorism). It offers a cynical and satirical account of how stereotyping and over-generalizing can be the con-sequences of waging war against bugs in space or, for the purposes of the present discussion, for learning that there might be terrorists in our midst.

The responses of the blogger-witnesses show that we some-times do more than watch. Sometimes witnesses help generate the terror that we are subject to and a terror that we impose on others.

Conclusion: 24 and a Passion for the Real

> Every terrorist wants something. Every terrorist needs
> something. Identifying what those needs and wants are
> can help you get information. Although you may know the
> terrorist organization's stated platform and objectives, you
> may not know what the individual in front of you seeks.
> You may also not have time to find out … If you are running
> out of time – as is often the case at CTU – find out what they
> want and then determine if giving it to them is a worth-
> while option. (*Counterterrorism Unit Operations Manual*)[70]

A fascinating article written by film producer Judd Aptow in October 2005, well before the Mumbai attacks, demonstrates the
links between celebrity and terrorism with sharp clarity.[72] Aptow
writes that he is concerned by the prevalence and aggression of tabloidized celebrity media, and that he is equally concerned about
how celebrities manipulate that media. He cites as an example the
relationship between Tom Cruise and Katie Holmes and the considerable media attention they receive. He argues, however, that
the witnesses of this celebrity media circus are hardly to blame.
Indeed, he thinks 9/11 is to blame:

> I think 9/11 is the cause of all of this. People are more freaked
> out than they can say out loud. If we all talked about how
> scared we are that someone is going to nuke a city, or blow
> up the electric grid, or whatever nightmarish thing you can
> think of as you close your eyes before you go to sleep, then
> none of us would be able to leave the house or go to work.
> The celebrity obsession is a fantastic distraction from an-
> thrax fears. I would rather read about Angelina Jolie and
> Brad Pitt than sit around wondering how bad the next at-
> tack will be in the United States. Maybe the terrorists feel
> the need to top their last atrocity and aren't going to do any-
> thing until they can make that happen.[73]

I want to conclude this chapter by suggesting that *terrorism is already celebritized*. Terrorism is so interwoven into notions of celeb-

rity, theater, and witnessing that it is challenging to distinguish the ways that it is conceptually and ontologically different to celebrity. Throughout this chapter I have prefaced each section with a quote from *The Official CTU Operations Manual* – a fictional user manual for new agents admitted to the Los Angeles branch of the "Counterterrorism Unit" as featured in the hit television show *24*. This fictional operations manual is presented and designed to look *real*. It is labeled and stamped with official-looking insignia of the CTU and the federal government, and on the cover it declares that one may read it only with a "minimum level 3 security clearance". The glossy book is housed in a solid, cardboard box. Upon opening the box the reader is immediately faced with an official looking warning: "STOP. CLASSIFIED MATERIAL. EYES ONLY … PROCEEDING WITHOUT APPROPRIATE CLEARANCE CONSITUTES A FEDERAL CRIME PUNISHABLE BY UP TO 25 YEARS IMPRISONMENT". This warning is followed by a return address to which the manual must be sent if found.

The television show *24* features all of the elements of a terror theater and all of the features of celebrity terrorism – the fictional terrorists they chase are household names in the fictional terror war depicted in *24*; the locations where attacks are planned are often major population centers and the terrorist conspiracy sometimes leads to the highest echelons of government. Even the agents take on a celebritized status, most notably through Jack Bauer, the sometimes renegade, breaks-the-rules-when-the-rules-are-unjust, agent extraordinaire. The entire program is a symbolic tribute to the post-9/11 world and a powerful illustration of how terrorism is already celebritized. A dedicated audience of followers was assured as soon as the show was conceived given the nature, structure and so-called *reality* of the post-9/11 world.

This dedicated audience, like many other witnesses of terrorism, are pursuing what Žižek has described as a *passion for the real*. 9/11 was – after many years of waiting –[74] a real and powerful event, but it eventually dissipated and partly vanished from most news programming. More representations of terrorism were needed to fill this void; 9/11 had generated a renewed lust for reality, a lust that had been temporarily satisfied by the reality television fad. Artifacts like the fictional counterterrorism operations manual and the television show *24* – and other tele-visual and screen artifacts in the post-9/11 world – have worked as temporary relief, providing encounters with 9/11 and terrorism as we lay in wait for the next *real* event.

This passion for the real does not end with *24*. As I will show in the remaining chapters of this book this passion can be found in many locations in the post-9/11 popular, tele-visual and screen cultural world.

Part II

9/11 as Popular Culture and Pornography

4.

Representing Terrorism
Re-animating Post-9/11 New York City

In all the television coverage, time and time again, not a voiceover, but an image behind all the reports and discussions, as if to show, again and again, to anyone who hadn't seen it yet, that this was real.[1]

The truth is that right after 9/11 I had a pin [of the American flag]. Shortly after 9/11, particularly because we're talking about the Iraq war, that became a substitute for I think true patriotism, which is speaking out on issues that are of importance to our national security ... I decided I won't wear that pin on my chest ... Instead, I'm going to try to tell the American people what I believe will make this country great, and hopefully that will be a testament to my patriotism (Barack Obama, October 2007).

Post-9/11 NYC

The absence of the Twin Towers from the post-9/11 New York City skyline posed a number of dilemmas for the creators and producers of television shows and movies that were "symbolically" set in New York City after 9/11. Whilst the World Trade Center towers had been destroyed, editors in studio lots in California faced the prospect of the late 2001 ratings season commencing with stock reels of New York City that prominently featured the Towers prior to 9/11. This posed an odd dilemma for the producers of television shows such as *Friends, Sex and the City,* and *Spin City,* programs in which the Twin Towers often appeared as a backdrop and a powerful signifier of being in New York City. The response seemed universal – the Twin Towers must be removed from the tele-visual pop-cultural locations. They needed to be purged, exorcized and air-brushed out of the shot. But by airbrushing out the Towers, the producers have purged post-9/11 television of more than just the steel and concrete of the iconic buildings. This purging is powerful, a little odd, and deeply symbolic. In order to recover perhaps some space – and some forgetting, if only temporary – was needed. But the missing Towers also represented a missing terror, a missing city. It was as though the creators and producers of some post-9/11 television believed that the world's viewers would have no stomach for seeing images of a pre-9/11 New York City – a city that in many respects no longer existed. Perhaps the problem lies in how the destruction of the Twin Towers was witnessed – live on TV, in real-time, as heinous, immediate and real violence. It was ugly, sickening, horrific, terrifying. Yet it was also difficult to look away.

Few representations of New York City in television programs were as intriguing as the representations in post-9/11 episodes of *Friends.* As such, I single out these episodes for special attention. The relationships between 9/11 and programs such as *Family Guy, American Dad, The Simpsons, How I Met Your Mother, The West Wing* and *24* are – for the most part – less problematic than the relationships between 9/11 and post-9/11 episodes of *Friends.* They should be viewed as special and serve as a case study for understanding the meanings and consequences of 9/11 in post-9/11 tele-visual popular culture.

In this chapter I will explore the representations of trauma, New York City, 9/11, terrorism, popular culture, fiction and reality in post-9/11 episodes of *Friends.* Terrorism and 9/11 is – paradoxically – both *present* (as part of the narrative backdrop, in set and wardrobe design) and *absent* (ignored, irrelevant, missing, or perhaps forgotten). I suggest that this uncanny presence-absence is a vehicle through which terrorism is represented (and *re*-represented) in *Friends* and where images of the city are imagined (and *re*-imagined) in a world that can be indefinitely described as post-9/11. I am assisted in this task by a variety of social theorists that include Slavoj Žižek, Zygmunt Bauman, Erich Fromm and others. Their work opens a space in which I seek to locate this chapter.

Watching *Friends* after 9/11

Friends introduced the world to six so-called "coffee house crowd" New Yorkers – Ross, Rachel, Monica, Chandler, Phoebe and Joey.[2] These six characters soon became pop-cultural icons. Women – and men – during the 1990s would visit hair salons and request "The Rachel". Funny-man Chandler introduced the world to the comedic prefix "Could I be anymore [insert noun/adjective]?" And womanizer Joey's well-known pick-up line – "how *you* doin'" – became an often heard joke. The creators and producers of *Friends* wanted to capture what it meant to be 20-something in Manhattan's apparently sexually promiscuous café culture and soon the situation-comedy became one of the world's most watched television programs.[3] Shortly before the commencement of series eight of *Friends*, 19 hijackers seized control of four passenger airplanes and slammed one into each of the Twin Towers in New York City, one into the Pentagon in Washington DC and a fourth crashed in a field in Shanksville, Pennsylvania. It is difficult to overstate the impact of these attacks in New York City and the reverberations felt throughout the world. Surely, what it meant to be a New Yorker had changed forever. Because of this I was surprised that when season eight commenced little had changed in the Manhattan of the eccentric and promiscuous characters in *Friends*. Perhaps it was my subjective position as a student of terrorism and, later, an academic and lecturer that led to my expectation that the changes witnessed in New York's skyline would be reflected in pop-cultural representations of New York City and – by extension – in the ways that New York and terrorism would be represented in our imaginations.

In many respects, however, the consequences of terrorism and 9/11 were absent from the post-9/11 episodes of *Friends*. Yet, despite this absence, 9/11 was not forgotten. It was there – in set design, in wardrobe decisions, in artwork, in tributes. No one spoke about it, no one was grieving, but it had happened – 9/11 had happened. In these ways I suggest that this absence was accompanied by a paradoxical presence – a type of presence-absence. I argue that this presence-absence represents an indecisive moment in *Friends*. If this was a moment of denial and forgetfulness then it was also a moment of trauma and of what psychoanalysts might call a "fetishistic disavowal".[4] I will explore this point in more detail later in this chapter, but for the moment I want to suggest that this disavowal might make it possible to view post-9/11 *Friends* as another in a series of what Žižek describes as *paranoiac fantasies*.[5] The paranoiac fantasy in post-9/11 *Friends* takes the form of a Manhattan where everyday life continues without fear and anxiety and without terror. Could post-9/11 *Friends* be, as Žižek posits, another in a series of consumable products that are deprived of their malignant properties? – "coffee without caffeine, cream without fat, beer without alcohol ... virtual sex as sex without sex, the Colin Powell doctrine of warfare without casualties ... as warfare without warfare".[6] I am tempted to argue that post-9/11 *Friends* sits well in this list of consumables as *New York without the terror* – a city without the insecurity.

It is perhaps in this context that we can best understand recent psychiatric diagnoses of "Truman Show syndrome" where those afflicted come to believe that their world "was slightly unreal" as if they were "the eponymous hero in the film *The Truman Show*".[7] Žižek seems to have predicted this in his conceptualization of *The Truman Show* as "the *ultimate* American paranoiac fantasy".[8] For Žižek "The ultimate American paranoiac fantasy is that of an individual living in ... a consumerist paradise, who suddenly starts to suspect that the world he is living in is a fake, a spectacle staged to convince him that he is living in a real world, while all the people around him are in fact actors and extras in a gigantic show".[9] The "underlying experience" of movies such as *The Truman Show* is "that the late-capitalist consumerist ... paradise is ... in a way unreal".[10] Žižek argues that the "same "derealization" of the horror went on after the WTC collapse".[11] The derealization of horror is a key feature of post-9/11 episodes of *Friends*. These episodes represented a routine of absence, forgetting, and amnesia. But this amnesia was not total. As Prager suggests, trauma is sometimes observed as a "paradoxical preservation of traumatic pasts into the present".[12] So whilst in constructing the narrative of post-9/11 Friends there were attempts to repress 9/11, the gestures, representations, presences and absences preserve and perhaps pay homage to Manhattan's traumatic past.

As an avid viewer of *Friends*, I was confronted with these dilemmas after 9/11 as it appeared that the program's producers and creators had not incorporated the 9/11 attacks into the narrative of series eight. How was I to understand the meaning of *Friends* after 9/11 when the Manhattan that the show depicted no longer existed? Had the characters repressed the events of 9/11? Were they in denial? Or were they the brave and resilient New Yorkers that could be seen in media images working together in the immediate aftermath of 9/11, sifting through rubble, comforting each other, looking for friends and family? Perhaps post-9/11 episodes of *Friends* were testimony that New York really had changed, that New Yorkers had been united by international terrorism and that the spirit of their communities would be strong and resilient.

It took many weeks for the smoke and debris to settle after 9/11 – but the Manhattan of *Friends* seemed immune. But this fictional Manhattan remained haunted by the specter of 9/11 – the initially hidden representations of 9/11 in the post-9/11 episodes, representations that I will explore later in this chapter, are evidence of this haunting. It was as though two parallel worlds – a fictional Manhattan and a real Manhattan – were collapsing into one. As a viewer of *Friends* and a witness of 9/11 in real-time on my television, what I sensed in the post-9/11 episodes was the potential, the likelihood and the danger of 9/11 occurring right in front of my eyes. It was as though I was waiting for the planes to strike. 9/11 in the post-9/11 episodes was – as Bauman might argue – *the iceberg in the city*.

For Bauman the psyche of Westerners is permanently scarred with what he dubs the "Titanic Syndrome".[13] The "Titanic Syndrome" represents the "horror" of falling through the "wafer-thin crust" of civilization into the icy uncertainty of nothingness.[14] It represents the contours of our forever precarious and vulnerable existences and the threats, risks and dangers that we try not to think about in our day-to-day lives. According to Bauman the iceberg is "silent", always outside of plain view, always lurking below the surface, and always devastating.[15] But the horror of the Titanic story, according to Bauman, does not come from the iceberg. Rather, the horror comes from the spectacle of the luxurious liner where the catastrophe appears and matters most – it is here that people were killed and the affluent comforts of the leisure liner were driven to the cold and murky depths of the ocean. The horror comes with the *possibility* that at any moment the most relaxed and comfortable surroundings can become the most dangerous place on Earth.

This is what I mean when I say that 9/11 was the iceberg in the city in the post-9/11 episodes of *Friends*. It was a world where the viewer *knows* that 9/11 has occurred, yet there was no evidence of destruction, smoke, death and debris. 9/11 was the seventh friend, even though it did not appear in the credits. Post-9/11 *Friends* can be viewed as a location for reconciling and negotiating divergent and conflicting images of New York City and for understanding the new coordinates of insecurity and precariousness of life in the city even if the fear, dread and danger were buffed out, glossed over and desperately hidden behind the fiction of the pop-cultural landscape.

Popular Culture and Hidden Meaning

Finding hidden meanings in popular culture is, perhaps, nothing new (of which Freud's Oedipus complex, and his associated examination of Oedipus Rex, is but one example).[16] Fromm argued that drama has always played a significant role in the function of everyday life and that humankind craves the opportunity to experience – as participants or in the audience – the "dramatization of the fundamental problems of human existence" and an "acting out of the very same problems which are thought out in philosophy and theology".[17] Fromm added:

> What is left of such dramatization of life in modern culture? Almost nothing. Man hardly ever gets out of the realm of man-made conventions and things, and hardly ever breaks through the surface of his routine ... If there is a fire, or a car collision in a big city, scores of people will gather and watch. Millions of people are fascinated daily by reportings of crimes and by detective stories. They religiously go to movies in which crime and passion are the two central themes. All this interest and fascination is not simply an expression of bad taste and sensationalism, *but of a deep longing for a dramatization of ultimate phenomena of human existence*, life and death, crime and punishment, the battle between man and nature.[18]

Fromm's statement as reproduced above should resonate with post-9/11 pop-culture and media audiences. 9/11 was – and continues to be – one of the most tele-visually viewed events in history. These acts of terrorism have had alarming consequences that include war, torture, bigotry and racism, Hollywood movies, counter-culture documentarians, conspiracy theories and a forever changed New York City skyline and city-scape. Amongst these signposts of post-9/11 culture sit the routine and ritualistic aspects of popular tele-visual culture that includes news and current affairs, television series (such as *The West Wing* which explicitly depicted the events of 9/11) and situation comedies (such as *Sex and the City* and *Friends* which did not depict 9/11).

Perhaps this is why post-9/11 episodes of *Friends* seemed so odd to me. There was not – on the surface – a culture of remembering in these episodes. The effect of this was a kind of *representation and image of terrorism in reverse*. Instead of the flaming Twin Towers, the Towers were simply no longer there – gone but not destroyed. Where once, Fromm argued, drama featured the cathartic playing out of fear, anxiety, love and desire through "high artistic and metaphysical" expression, drama soon found expression in "crude" social trends, routines and rituals and produced no "cathartic effect" at all.[19] Certainly, there was little in the way of a post-9/11 catharsis in *Friends*. Where had the "absolute event" of 9/11 vanished too?[20] Why was it purged? Could this be what Baudrillard was talking about when he described 9/11 as a non-event?

Trauma and Representations of New York City and Terrorism

During and following 9/11 millions of people became overnight television and news media junkies. According to Rob Hirst, CNN's 24-hour news channel regularly attracted between 600000 and 800000 viewers during peak viewing periods prior to 9/11.[21] Following the attacks CNN's news broadcast regularly attracted three million viewers during peak hours. However, as Hirst argues:

> If ratings are any indication, though, most Americans are about as interested in their devolving international conflict [in Afghanistan] as they've traditionally been in the ballot box, remaining resolutely glued to sitcoms like *Friends* (which regularly pulls in over 30 million viewers).[22]

Interest in *Friends* had waned in the series that had aired just prior to 9/11. Series eight – which began airing shortly after 9/11 – saw the sitcom experience renewed popularity. As Szymanek argues, "It was right around 9/11 that it [*Friends*] entered its 8th season and it was once again cool to be a fan, but also comforting and even healing in the face of tragedy to know they've been here all the time".[23] It was through *Friends* – this Manhattan-based sitcom – that the trauma in Manhattan on 9/11 could be managed and perhaps one day suppressed, denied or forgotten. Or, if this proved to be too ambitious, *Friends* could be a place for the healing to begin.

Most explorations of the social and cultural meanings of trauma have tended to focus on the immediate physical and emotional consequences of traumatic events – how people have lived with physical injury and emotional scarring, how sites of trauma have been forever infused with a traumatic gloss, how we act out in the face of trauma and anxiety, and how images of trauma can haunt us and continue to inflict damage and casualties long after the disaster has passed.[24] Amongst this literature, the physical and psychological consequences of trauma are rightly privileged. Through the physical and psychological change it sparks, trauma has often been viewed as *cathartic*. I am particularly interested in how traumatic events – especially terrorism – are incorporated into social and cultural narratives. When series eight of *Friends* began such a social and cultural narrative was lacking. If this was the end of the story perhaps there would be no need for this chapter – it was, after all, a fictional Manhattan that the characters in *Friends* inhabited and, in time, I would have been comfortable viewing *Friends* knowing that 9/11 had been purged. I could have concluded that in the fictional world of *Friends* there was no 9/11, no death and destruction, and no trauma.

However, it was at this point that I became aware that the social and cultural accounts of trauma that emphasized the catharsis of trauma were inadequate to describe what was happening in post-9/11 *Friends*. Barthes in his account of the traumatic image, for example, explored what it means to witness the real event as an image – in some respects Barthes highlighted the problem of authenticity in experiencing trauma in images.[25] Similar dilemmas have been tackled by Žižek and Baudrillard.[26] But these accounts rely on real images of violence and horror for understanding trauma. But what if the trauma is not readily visible even when witnesses know it is there? How should we understand the images of post-9/11 New York City that confronted the viewer of post-9/11 episodes of *Friends* when 9/11 had been purged – airbrushed out of the shot before a traumatic reaction could be generated?

Žižek argues that "forgetting" plays an important role in any attempt to understand traumatic violence.[27] He considers how witnesses can go about their lives after watching spectacular violence:

> Would the watcher be able to continue going on as usual? Yes, but only if he or she were able to somehow forget – in an act which suspended symbolic efficiency – what had been witnessed. This forgetting entails a gesture of what is called *fetishist disavowal*: 'I know, but I don't want to know that I know, so I don't know'. I know it, but I refuse to fully assume the consequences of this knowledge, so that I can continue acting as if I don't know it.[28]

Such *fetishistic disavowal* was played out again and again in the post-9/11 episodes of *Friends*. It was played out so quickly and subtly that for many viewers of *Friends* it would have surely gone unnoticed. But, despite its disavowal, it was there – *terrorism* and *9/11* was there. It was captured, represented and animated, and then re-represented and re-animated in the Manhattan of Ross, Rachel, Monica, Chandler, Phoebe and Joey.[29]

The 9/11 terrorist attacks were not simply repressed, denied or forgotten. Whilst the characters were not covered in soot, ash and dust, and none had been rendered hospitalized or homeless, 9/11 was still represented in particular ways in the narratives of post-9/11 *Friends*. It appeared as a changed storyline in an early episode of series eight, as artwork in *Central Perk* café, as messages on a whiteboard attached to the front door of Chandler and Joey's apartment, and as clothing worn by Joey and Rachel. The trauma of 9/11 was visible in the backgrounds, wardrobe and artifacts of post-9/11 *Friends*. This contradictory presence and absence is evidence of a traumatic reaction – a reaction perhaps shared by all witnesses of terrorism both near and far from terrorisms' *flashpoint*.[30]

Perhaps, as Žižek[31] argues, trauma always evades clear recollection or remembering and therefore cannot be adequately incorporated into the symbolic narratives of everyday life in *Friends*:

> "trauma" designates a shocking encounter which, precisely, DISTURBS this immersion into one's life-world, a violent intrusion of something which doesn't fit in … Man is not simply overwhelmed by the impact of the traumatic encounter … but is able … to counteract its destabilizing impact by spinning out intricate symbolic cobwebs.[32]

Maybe this is why the writers and producers of *Friends* could find only a limited role – a role restricted to background imagery and set and wardrobe design – for the trauma of the 9/11 terrorist attacks in their continuing narratives of the lives of six supposedly typical people living in Manhattan. For the most part, it would seem that the most significant event in the history of New York's most tele-visually hyperknown borough had little role in the idyllic lives of Ross, Rachel, Monica, Chandler, Phoebe and Joey in the "traumascape" of Manhattan.[33] Maybe ignorance is bliss.

Indeed, Toby Miller suggests that "Being Ignorant" was an important part of living in Manhattan.[34] He argues that cosmopolitan New Yorkers could not have been further removed from the violence that raged throughout the rest of the world or the terrible vengeance exacted by the United States military following the attacks. According to Miller, 9/11 was so significant because of the "high premium immediately set on the lives of Manhattan residents and the rarefied discussion of how to commemorate the high-altitude towers".[35] After 9/11, Manhattan could no longer be viewed as just a cultural, financial, fashionable and sexual metropolis – we are now only too aware that it is also a terrorist target. Perhaps even a site for violent blowback. Native-American academic Ward Churchill takes this argument a step further.[36] He argues that the workers in the Twin Towers were natural and legitimate targets of international terrorism.

> True enough, they were civilians of a sort. But innocent? Gimme a break. They formed a technocratic corps at the

heart of America's global financial empire ... the "mighty engine of profit" to which the military dimensions of U.S. policy has always been enslaved – and they did so both willingly and knowingly.[37]

Zygmunt Bauman similarly argues that:

It was the actions of the United States together with its various satellites, like the World Bank, the International Monetary Fund and the World Trade Organization, that [quoting Arundhati Roy] 'promoted subsidiary developments, dangerous sub-products such as nationalism, religious fanaticism, fascism, and of course terrorism, advancing marching step in step with the neoliberal project of globalization'.[38]

This opens an alarming Pandora's Box. Could it be that the characters in *Friends* were the natural and legitimate targets of international terrorism? If they were, then perhaps so were Carrie, Miranda, Samantha and Charlotte and all the crew from the Manhattan depicted in *Sex and the City*.[39] Much like their fellow New Yorkers – those six friends spending their days drinking coffee at Central Perk – the Manhattan of the women of *Sex and the City* was not subject to the trauma of 9/11. It seemed that Carrie and co were not only immune to New York City's high crime, gang violence and – for the most part – a host of sexually transmitted diseases, but also from "the other star of the show," post-9/11 New York City.[40]

Some Perspective

Perhaps I need to regain some perspective. Perhaps I have ignored a more simple explanation for 9/11's presence-absence in the post-9/11 storyline of *Friends*. After all, *Friends*, unlike *Sex and the City*, was not performed or filmed in New York City. It was filmed in Studio City, California. The set was a simulation of a café and an apartment in Manhattan. Perhaps this was why the writers and producers of *Friends* could not envision a post-9/11 Manhattan café culture. The New York City of *Friends* was, both literally and figuratively, an "Imaginary New York":

The New York City within which *Friends* was set is an imaginary place in the American psyche where some of our most powerful mythologies intersect. One of the most resonant myths features New York as a place where young people who might not feel comfortable in their home towns can find community and blossom, just like these sitcom characters.[41]

The imaginary dimensions of the New York City in *Friends* means that the program was deeply absent and alienated from Manhattan, right down to the fictitious coffee house constructed out of images from coffee houses in Greenwich Village. *Friends* was an idyllic simulation of Manhattan.[42]

The presence-absence of 9/11 in *Friends* mirrors the presence-absence of the Twin Towers – their disappearance still casts a large shadow over the streets of New York. The gaping hole in the ground at Ground Zero is a scar of sorts – albeit one embodied by an absence – on the New York skyline. In some respects, it is difficult to sustain the argument that the Twin Towers no longer exist. It may be that the Twin Towers are more visible, present and well-known now that they are gone.

Accounting for Post-9/11 *Friends*

I am tempted to describe the analysis of *Friends* that I undertake in this chapter as a *narrative analysis*. A narrative analysis, in some conceptions, always has something to do with "words". The analysis that I undertake here, however, has less to do with "words" than images, symbols and *absences* of words. According to Lee et al., "Narrative is a universal genre of both oral language and written texts".[43] In such a view the analysis in this chapter could not really be said to constitute "narrative" analysis. Yet, Riessman's understanding of "narrative" provides a way of expanding on narrower definitions. She argued that narrative analysis "takes as its object" the "story".[44] Indeed, words do not structure narratives as much as human life is already "narratively structured".[45]

As such, the analysis that I undertake in this chapter is a form of narrative analysis, albeit one based on images, symbols and the absences of words. I am inspired in this endeavor by Elizabeth Grosz:

A text, whether book, paper, film, painting, or building, can be thought of as a kind of *thief in the night*. Furtive, clandestine, and always complex, it steals ideas from all around, from its own milieu and history, and better still from its outside, and disseminates them elsewhere. It is not only a conduit for the circulation of ideas, as knowledges or truths, but a passage or point of transition from one (social) stratum or space to another.[46]

Post-9/11 episodes of *Friends* – the sitcom that was filmed in Los Angeles, symbolically set in New York City, and incorporated 9/11 narratives without discussion, talk and words – embody such a "thief in the night". In this way, *Friends* is not a "repository of knowledges or truths" or a space where information is stored, but rather a "process of scattering thoughts; scrambling terms, concepts, and practices; forging linkages; becoming a form of action".[47] Grosz has explored at length the meaning of the body in the traumatic everydayness of the city-scape where "The city is a product not simply of the muscles and energy of the body, but of the conceptual and reflective possibilities of consciousness itself".[48] Grosz's work – when used alongside the work of various social theorists – opens a space for accounts of 9/11, New York City and Manhattan and the "War on Terror" that are imagined, fictional, anxiety-induced, virtual, hyperreal, corporeal, real, or visible and perhaps even absent.

To explore the 9/11 narratives in *Friends* I watched the full ten seasons from beginning to end over several weeks in early 2008 and reviewed some episodes additional times as I searched for more specific information. I observed the differences in how images of New York City were used in series eight, nine and ten – the post-9/11 episodes – when compared to the first seven seasons. As I watched I took detailed notes and watched the insightful bonus features that accompany each season on DVD. I paid particular attention to the backgrounds and sets and the stock footage of New York City in the opening and closing credits and in transitions between scenes. I set out to document how the 9/11 terrorist attacks and post-9/11 New York City were incorporated into the post-9/11 episodes of *Friends*.

Fragments of 9/11 in *Friends*

When I watched post-9/11 episodes of *Friends* in this way I began to see 9/11 as playing a significant role. An example of this can be found in the use of stock footage of New York City in both the pre- and post-9/11 episodes. In series one through seven, the images of New York City in the opening credits and scene transitions routinely featured the Twin Towers from various angles ranging from a broad and distant view of the New York skyline to an up-close, almost street level view. Occasionally the Twin Towers could be seen in the background of images of the apartment block where Rachel, Monica, Chandler and Joey (but not Ross and Phoebe – they lived elsewhere in Manhattan) lived. The first thing that the audiences of post-9/11 episodes witnessed with the commencement of series eight was a different set of stock footage of images of New York City used in the opening credits and in transitions between scenes. In series eight, nine and ten there were no images of the Twin Towers in any of the skyline images of New York. This may not seem remarkable at first glance, but when one considers that the images of New York used in *Friends* were likely drawn from generic reels of stock footage, finding images of the Manhattan skyline that did not feature the Twin Towers may have been difficult. Certainly the number of available images would have been significantly reduced. The producers of *Sex and the City* similarly expunged all images and references to the Twin Towers from the show. In the early episodes of series eight of *Friends* there were also a number of broad and abstract references to 9/11, American culture and New Yorker identity. Importantly, the creators of *Friends* signaled a new signpost in post-9/11 television by dedicating the first episode of season eight – "The One After 'I Do'" – "to the people of New York City".[49] This was quickly followed by a changed storyline for episode three of season eight – "The One Where Rachel Tells".[50] As Monica and Chandler left for their honeymoon the script originally called for Chandler to make an inappropriate remark about a bomb in the airport.[51] Not funny in a post-9/11 world.

There were two key spaces in the background set of *Friends* that were used to pay tribute to the people of New York and the United States in the first post-9/11 season. The first of these spaces was the wall behind the famous couch where the *Friends* crew sat in their favorite coffee house – Central Perk. The artwork on this wall was changed every two or three episodes. After 9/11 this artwork sometimes depicted American flags, images of "Uncle Sam", and caricatures of the Statue of Liberty. In the pre-9/11 series the viewer was more likely to see artwork featuring mundane images of animals, flowers and murals of shapes and color. The second space was a whiteboard that hung on the front door of Joey and Chandler's apartment. The whiteboard was used throughout the *Friends* series for notes, images, and messages. After 9/11 this space was used to pay tribute to New Yorkers and their emergency services. The following table depicts how these spaces were used in series eight of *Friends*. Also depicted in this table are miscellaneous representations of 9/11 and post-9/11 New York City in this series.

Many of the references to 9/11 were sporadic, occasional and more likely the result of idiosyncratic wardrobe and set design decisions rather than narrative planning. But they were there for all viewers to see. At times the changing artwork in the background of scenes filmed in Central Perk depicted images of American culture – Uncle Sam, the Statue of Liberty, and American flags. The whiteboard at one point contained the doodled words "One New York. 1 People". At another point the whiteboard contained the letters "FDNY" (Fire Department, New York). On three separate occasions in series eight characters could be seen wearing FDNY t-shirts. Another post-9/11 change could be seen in a poster behind the fridge in Joey and Chandler's apartment. For several seasons the space behind their fridge had been filled with a cartoonish map of Manhattan. Eight episodes into series eight this image was replaced by an American flag. What this had to do with post-9/11 New York is unclear. But Hirst writes of being in Los Angeles immediately following 9/11:

> The US flag is everywhere, sold in its thousands by those guys at intersections who clean your windscreens whether you like it or not. It hangs from private verandahs and office windows, and it's stuck to the bonnets and boots of countless Chevvies, Hondas and Beemers.[52]

Episode	Air date	Whiteboard	Artwork in Central Perk	Miscellaneous references
1	27-Sep-01	- (not visible)	- (not visible)	Episode dedicated to the people of New York City
2	4-Oct-01	-	Painting of fruit	-
3	11-Oct-01	Sketch of Empire State Building	-	Changed storyline – Chandler's "bomb joke"
4	18-Oct-01	I ♥ New York	-	-
5	25-Oct-01	Sketch of mushroom	Painting of fruit	-
6	1-Nov-01	-	- (distorted)	"FDNY" t-shirt - Joey
7	8-Nov-01	Sketch of robots	Painting of chair	-
8	15-Nov-01	Sketch of US flag on moon	Painting of Statue of Liberty/Flag	*American flag near fridge
9	22-Nov-01	The phrase - "One New York, 1 People"	-	*American flag near fridge
10	6-Dec-01	The acronym "FDNY"	Painting of Statue of Liberty/Flag	*American flag near fridge
11	13-Dec-01	Sketch of bird and flowers	Christmas wreath	"FDNY" t-shirt - Rachel
12	10-Jan-02	Sketch of Sun/Moon hybrid	Painting of white flower	"Capt. Billy Burke" t-shirt
13	17-Jan-02	Sketch of a train	An American flag	*American flag near fridge
14	31-Jan-02	Sketch of a hockey-goalie	Abstract painting of a bulldog	*American flag near fridge
15	7-Feb-02	Sketch of a motorcycle	Valentine's Day wreath	*American flag near fridge
16	28-Feb-02	face	Painting of a cow	*American flag near fridge
17	7-Mar-02	-	Painting of the Statue of Liberty	*American flag near fridge
18	28-Mar-02	-	-	*American flag near fridge
19	4-Apr-02	-	Painting of "Uncle Sam"	*American flag near fridge
20	25-Apr-02	- (distorted)	-	*American flag near fridge
21	2-May-02	-	Painting of "Uncle Sam"	*American flag near fridge
22	9-May-02	-	Painting of "Uncle Sam"	*American flag near fridge
23	16-May-02	-	-	*American flag near fridge
24	16-May-02	-	-	*American flag near fridge

Table 1: The Whiteboard, Artwork in *Central Perk* and miscellaneous representations of 9/11, terrorism and New York City in post-9/11 *Friends* (* permanent in post 9/11 episodes from episode eight of series eight until the program's conclusion after ten seasons).

Hirst argues that for some this flag-waving was part of the grieving process, but for others, it represented a dark hostility towards the world outside of the US. This hostility was embodied by bumper-stickers and t-shirts that were fused and linked to images of the US flag – "IT'S BUTT-KICKING TIME"; "DON'T FUCK WITH US. WE FUCK BACK".[53] This may be evidence of a post-9/11 world where a lust for nationalistic symbolism and the desire to stake one's devotion to the symbolic tribalization of nationhood could take hold as a renewed devotion to "blood" and "soil".[54]

It is not clear which wielding of the flag was present in post-9/11 episodes of *Friends*. But perhaps the post-9/11 appearance of a permanent American flag in *Friends* can shed light on the controversy surrounding Barack Obama's failure to don an American flag lapel pin in the early stages of the 2007/2008 Presidential election campaign. Barack Obama moved against this political routine early in his Presidential campaign because he believed that the American flag had become a substitute for "true patriotism".[55] In a statement from his campaign offices it was declared "We all revere the flag, but Senator Obama believes that being a patriot is about more than a symbol".[56]

Locating 9/11 in *Friends*

The visible presence-absence of 9/11 in *Friends* – represented by artwork, notes on whiteboards, clothing and American flags – finds an unstable footing in the time and space coordinates of the post-9/11 episodes. The producers and directors of *Friends* had always attempted to keep the program's schedule, as much as possible, in line with "real" world chronology. For example, series eight began airing on 27 September 2001. The Halloween episode aired to correspond with the "real world" Halloween. The Thanksgiving episode corresponded with Thanksgiving and the Christmas episode aired shortly before the show went off air over Christmas before returning in January. In February the Valentine's Day episode was aired. Naturally this narrative was constantly broken by the beginning and end of the US ratings seasons. So whilst the audience can imagine that when the season starts the temporality of the in-world narrative corresponds roughly with the temporal conditions outside of the world of *Friends*, at some point during the between-season breaks this chronology becomes incongruent. How is the viewer to understand the day before the first post-9/11 series begins? The last episode of series seven featured Chandler's and Monica's wedding. According to the *Friends* temporal narrative the first episode of series eight is the next day despite season seven ending in May and season eight beginning in September, shortly after 9/11. As such, the lives of the characters in *Friends* at the beginning of series eight corresponded with a "real" world period of mourning, horror and anxiety for large numbers of television audiences.

Why is this even important? I suggest it is important because it represents a crucial antagonism that is produced in most television programs that depict routine and everyday life. It is an antagonism of time and space. Is not 9/11 as an event of the same order? Massive and horrific terrorist attacks occurred in New York City on 11 September 2001 but it was – and is – witnessed across multiple configurations of time and space even as it was occurring. But where did 9/11 go in the fictional narrative of *Friends*? It was not, after all, totally absent. There were t-shirts, paintings and whiteboard doodles – all are testament to perhaps the most significant event in the lives of these six New Yorkers. The building where Monica, Rachel, Chandler and Joey live is a building in Manhattan located on the corner of Bedford and Grove – or at least that is the building where the producers would have the audience believe that they live. The Bedford-Grove intersection is a real intersection in Manhattan. As such, 9/11 would have caused more than a slight interruption to the everyday lives of these six friends. Perhaps if the show was to reach for a deeper reality, one of the characters could have died. Chandler would have been a likely candidate as he worked in a tall office building for a major international firm. Perhaps Ross – a Professor of Paleontology at New York University – was having breakfast with NYU colleagues at the time the planes struck, and perhaps these colleagues watched the events unfold on television together. Social theorist Toby Miller was an NYU Professor when 9/11 occurred – perhaps these NYU colleagues were having coffee together (perhaps at *Central Perk*) when they heard an explosion and smoke filled the Manhattan sky. Of course I can easily shake myself out of this fantasy – *Friends* was, in reality, filmed in Studio City, California.

But here is my dilemma. Every time I snap back to reality and remember that *Friends* is fiction no matter how real it seems something else shunts me out of this reality and absorbs me back into the fictitious world of these "everyday" New Yorkers. It was filmed in a studio in California no matter how well the show's creators simulate Manhattan. So why acknowledge 9/11 at all? Should viewers interpret the 9/11 references in post-9/11 episodes of *Friends* as a wholly Californian tribute? Or, perhaps the links to a post-9/11 time and space are not really there. Images of American flags,

Uncle Sam, and the Statue of Liberty are routine features of life in America (despite the appearance of an American flag in series one to seven being a rare occurrence). Yet, there was one representation of 9/11 that could not be denied when in episode twelve of season eight – titled "The One Where Joey Dates Rachel" – Joey casually lounges around his apartment wearing a t-shirt with the words "Capt. Billy Burke" on the chest.[57]

Captain Billy Burke has become a well-known heroic figure of the 9/11 terrorist attacks. Burke was a firefighter who perished in the Twin Towers when they collapsed. When Tower Two collapsed Captain Burke was on the 27th floor of Tower One. Captain Burke ordered his colleagues out of the Tower but remained in the burning building with Ed Beya, a quadriplegic man, and the man's friend, Abe Zelmanowitz. These three remained together, refusing to leave each other's side, as Tower One fell to the Manhattan streets below the World Trade Center.[58]

The reference to Billy Burke in post-9/11 *Friends* works to shatter the very fabric of reality in the fictional world of Ross, Rachel, Monica, Chandler, Phoebe and Joey. If all the gestures and representations of 9/11 in series eight could be chalked up to my situatedness, or perhaps my paranoia, the invoking and reanimating of the story of Billy Burke provided particularly compelling evidence that I was not jumping at shadows (at least not on this occasion). No longer can I say that the 9/11 references were more a product of idiosyncratic set and wardrobe decisions. This t-shirt would have been difficult to find, perhaps specially ordered and made, or perhaps it was sent by Captain Burke's colleagues for use in one of America's most popular sitcoms. Regardless of how the t-shirt found its way into post-9/11 *Friends*, it represented something quite different to a presence-absence. The t-shirt symbolically placed *Friends* in a post-9/11 world. It was real and, therefore, now, so was 9/11.

Conclusion: When it Hasn't Been Your Day, Week, Month or Even Your Year

Friends never really occupied a subversive political, social and cultural space. The program was designed to appeal to a mass audience and has regularly been aired on major US and global networks in so-called "prime-time" time slots. It remained one of the highest rating television shows in the US and Australia for most of its 10 years on air. But unlike its comedic counterpart *The Simpsons* and the cartoonish antics of Homer and Bart, *Friends* rarely attempted to politically subvert, fracture social and cultural boundaries, or engage in targeted social commentary (a space that even the light-treading *Family Ties* explored!).

In many respects the creators of *Friends* did not incorporate 9/11 into the program's narrative, but they did acknowledge the events of 9/11 through a variety of representations and gestures and by generating a paradoxical presence-absence for the 9/11 terrorist attacks. These representations and gestures were expressed through the use of American flags, images of the Statue of Liberty, images of Uncle Sam, FDNY t-shirts and the reference to Captain Billy Burke. These artifacts represent problematic *antagonisms of reality* in the narratives of the fictional Manhattan depicted in *Friends*. Certainly as a fictional television program it did not have to be *real*, so perhaps there is no dilemma. Then why choose a "real" apartment block for the characters to live in? Why employ various cultural icons representing New York and Manhattan? Why pay tribute to Captain Billy Burke? These questions are not easily explained away by an appeal to an unproblematic reality. As Zurawik argues: "As much as the series has been criticized for its lack of social reality in terms of diversity, cost of living, crime and gridlock, it was that very *lack of reality* ... that gave it a second life after 9/11. This was a New York where people loved each other and made babies, not a New York where hate-filled zealots crashed planes into towers".[59]

This "lack of reality" represents a moment of denial, forgetfulness and trauma – a "fetishist disavowal".[60] *We know but we don't want to know, so we pretend that we do not know.* As such, post-9/11 *Friends* takes its rightful place among the many products that are deprived of their malignant properties – the New York in post-9/11 *Friends* represents *New York without the terror* and, therefore, *New York City without its New Yorkness*. In this way, post-9/11 *Friends* joins *The Truman Show* as "the *ultimate* American paranoiac fantasy".[61] I suggest that the "underlying experience" of *Friends* is that post-9/11 New York City is, in a way, *unreal*.

Or perhaps I should once again shunt myself back to reality and adjust my perspective. Perhaps *Friends* represents a New York

City where people can again be ignorant. New York City may be an idyllic and glamorous setting for popular culture, but in a post-9/11 world it is a terrorist target. The post-9/11 episodes of *Friends* could also be viewed as a vain attempt at normalizing what was a catastrophic event that has induced deep anxieties in affluent city-dwelling witnesses. The Manhattan of Ross, Rachel, Monica, Chandler, Phoebe and Joey was a paranoid one. They feigned business as usual as the world collapsed around them – and we watched. Post-9/11 *Friends* was a symbolic location where the ills of the world were suspended – if only for half-an-hour per week. Despite this (or perhaps because of this), grim reality haunted the *Friends* set in Studio City, California. No longer was the Manhattan of *Friends* a place where the apparently promiscuous café-culture came to play, it was also a terrorist target. But hey, "Your mother warned you there'd be days like these".[62]

5.

They Were Created by Man …
and They Have a Plan
Subjective and Objective Violence
in *Battlestar Galactica* and the War on Terror

Since tragedy, comedy, and light comedy fail to please him precisely because of their perfection, he turns to farce. The same phenomenon is repeated in other spheres.[1]

All this has happened before, and all of it will happen again.[2]

Repetition and Farce in the "War on Terror"

Tele-visual cultures have played a significant role in representing the meanings and consequences of the 9/11 terrorist attacks. The re-imagined *Battlestar Galactica* (BSG) television series has been particularly influential in articulating a critical account of 9/11 and the so-called "War on Terror". BSG regularly attracted over two million viewers each week when it was first aired and it has been the impetus for a body of scholarly thought that should perhaps be described as *Battlestar Galactica Studies*.[3] More than anything, the re-imagined BSG is *about* 9/11. It is the story of the human race attempting to avoid an apocalypse at the hands of a race of robots called Cylons. Humans created Cylons to be a race of slaves, but they were self-aware and rebelled against their human masters. But this is only part of the story. There is a broader story with broader implications that belies both BSG and the "War on Terror". To understand the significance of this broader story I analyze in this chapter the re-imagined BSG with the aid of Žižek's theoretical accounts of "subjective" and "objective" violence. When BSG and the "War on Terror" are viewed through this theoretical lens we can better understand the significance and meanings of terrorist violence and maybe even provide a space from which to predict where the next 9/11 will come from. An enduring catch phrase from BSG, "All of this has happened before, and all of this will happen again", should be understood alongside Žižek's work on violence. In doing so we may also come to understand that when terrorist violence is allowed to "happen again", it does so first as tragedy, then as farce. The most important thing about the next 9/11 will be that it could have been prevented.

This chapter is ordered in the following way: first, I outline the theoretical distinctions that allow divergent realities of violence to emerge. These are described as *subjective* and *objective* violence. Second, I offer an account of the re-imagined *Battlestar Galactica* television series emphasizing representations of subjective and objective violence. I explore the ways that these representations interact with a world that can be indefinitely described as post-9/11. It is a world where the response to 9/11 is making another 9/11 more likely – *the first 9/11 was a tragedy, but the second one will be a farce.* As we wait and worry about the next terrorist disaster, BSG in a post-9/11 world reminds us that the next generation of terrorists will likely emerge from some familiar places and for some clear reasons. When this happens it will be a farce of repetition of the highest order. There is always hope of preventing terrorism but in the "War on Terror" we are bound to cycles of violence that ensure that the next catastrophic act of terrorism is not only a possibility, but a certainty.

Subjective and Objective Violence

Žižek's descriptions of the distinction between "subjective" and "objective" violence is prologued with a joke about a worker who was suspected by managers in his company of stealing from the factory where he worked.[4] Each night as the worker left the factory his wheelbarrow was carefully searched for any evidence that he was stealing. In turned out, however, that what the worker was stealing was wheelbarrows.

Žižek uses this joke to redirect our attention away from the most visible forms of violence that we encounter in contemporary society through the global media and in the everydayness of life. As witnesses of violence we – for very good reasons – focus on the most visible, brutal and vulgar acts. Murders, assaults, rapes, terrorism and war fill media spaces and induce deep anxieties. These, for Žižek, are moments of "subjective" violence. But, as witnesses to subjective violence, we must "learn to step back" and witness the systemic and symbolic "contours" of the contemporary world, contours that sustain and organize visible and brutal acts of violence.[5]

> We should learn to ... disentangle ourselves from the fascinating lure of this directly visible "subjective" violence, violence performed by a clearly identifiable agent. We need to perceive the contours of the background which generates such outbursts. A step back enables us to identify a violence that sustains our very efforts to fight violence and to promote tolerance.[6]

This background violence – or, "objective" violence – has two forms. The first is "symbolic" violence which takes shape through speech acts and forms.[7] The other is "systemic" violence which is "the often catastrophic consequences of the smooth functioning of our economic and political systems".[8] The distinction between subjective and objective violence underpins some of Žižek's earlier theorizing on violence as well. Of particular note in this theorizing is his descriptions of what he calls *repressive desublimation*.[9]

Repressive desublimation, for Žižek, involves a process through which the mediating influence of the ego (ego meaning in this context the socialized self) is symbolically deprived of its usual autonomy over human behaviour. An absent or underdeveloped ego may often be associated with people who do not effectively control their impulses and desires making them prone to outbursts of aggression and violence (ie: anti-social behaviour). In Žižek's view, when such aggression or violence occurs it may appear that the absent ego has paved the way for the compulsions of the *id*.[10] A close look may reveal, however, that something quite different has happened, that the active force in generating outbursts of aggression and violence is not the desires of the id, but the societal commands and permissions afforded by the *superego* (superego meaning in this context, our societal and cultural rule-following behaviours). Stated differently, repressive desublimation is the pathway through which outbursts of subjective violence are grounded in the societal conditions that make such outbursts possible. Examples of repressive desublimation are common in the social and cultural history of war and violence. An obvious example is the "Good Germans" of World War II. War time Germany was a place where anti-Semitism was not viewed as anti-social. Rather, it was a mark of being a good German; a German with Germany's social, cultural and economic interests at heart. Something similar was happening after 9/11. Critiques of the looming post-9/11 wars were often branded as unpatriotic as all "Good Americans" were called upon to show whether they were with America or with the terrorists. In this environment, some found anti-Muslim sentiment and action to be a way of demonstrating a powerful allegiance to America. Repressive desublimation permits surrender to aggressive and violent impulses and temptations to the extent that such a space is provided by the prevailing societal conditions.[11]

Perhaps the most relevant articulation of the distinction between subjective and objective violence is offered by Žižek in *The Parallax View* where he draws attention away from the subjective violence of the "war on terror" towards the background that made this violence inevitable. Žižek argues in a section exploring the meanings of the torture perpetrated by American soldiers in the notorious Abu Ghraib prison in Iraq:

> *recording* the humiliation with a camera, with the perpetrators *included* in the picture, their faces stupidly smiling alongside the naked and twisted bodies of the prisoners, is an integral part of the process, in stark contrast to the secrecy of Saddam's tortures … to anyone acquainted with the reality of the US way of life, the photos immediately brought to mind the obscene underside of US popular culture … The Abu Ghraib tortures are thus to be located in the series of obscene underground practices that sustain an ideological edifice.[12]

Žižek reflects on how the torture at Abu Ghraib so resembles the initiation ceremonies that take place across education, military and sporting institutions, and in gangs and secret societies throughout the US. These frat-house initiations too take on perverse sexual dimensions. In short, the subjective violence at Abu Ghraib reflects inherent desires and behaviours exhibited in day-to-day US life – the "theatre of cruelty" played out in US pop-culture and everyday life.[13]

In the post-9/11 world, the distinction between subjective and objective violence can have significant consequences. Through the outbursts of subjective violence on 9/11 governments and their militaries have built cases to launch wars in Iraq and Afghanistan, located, tortured and charged suspected terrorists,[14] and have carried out retributions against those deemed responsible for harboring and aiding terrorism. Identifying objective violence often means something quite different. These same governments and militaries have little interest in identifying the objective contours of subjective violence. To do so would leave many governments and militaries vulnerable to the same charge that they have leveled at those they deem "terrorists", a phenomenon that Chomsky once described as a "Culture of Terrorism".[15] Those who have pointed out that subjective violence does not take place in a vacuum, that there are systemic conditions that form the basis of oppression and exploitation without which subjective violence would not be possible, leave themselves open to charges of being "pro-terrorist", "unpatriotic" and perhaps even "loony leftist", to borrow a few that are thrown around talk-back radio and on the *Fox News* channel. In short, identifying objective violence can have consequences. Yet, identifying objective violence may also play an important role in preventing terrorism.

The differences between subjective and objective violence can be accounted for in many ways. For the purposes of this chapter, I am most interested in how subjective and objective violence appear as organizing principles for the "War on Terror" and the post-9/11 television series *Battlestar Galactica*. The subjective and objective violence represented in BSG mirrors the subjective and objective violence of the "War on Terror". This is not a coincidence. As Dudley argues:

> What a shock it was ... to see the new series [of BSG] emerge
> as a deliberate and uncompromising attempt to confront the
> aftermath of the September 11th attacks and the "war on
> terror". From its inception as a mini-series in which human-
> ity is all but wiped out in a sneak attack by a seemingly
> inhuman enemy, to its almost unrelievedly bleak portrait of
> a civilization trying to retain its fundamental values in the
> face of an ongoing threat – and often failing spectacularly –
> "Battlestar Galactica" has acted as nothing less than a kind
> of immersion therapy for post-9/11 America.[16]

BSG is viewing for the post-9/11 consumer. When I first watched
the re-imagined BSG it seemed that the creators even assumed that
their audience had witnessed the 9/11 terror attacks live on television.

Subjective and Objective Violence in *Battlestar Galactica*

BSG is the story of the human race on the verge of extinction
hurtling through space whilst being pursued by a race of human-
created machines called *Cylons*. What was believed to be the lone
surviving "battlestar" class spaceship – the *Galactica* – leads the
civilian fleet of ships towards the mythical human colony called
Earth. The re-imagined BSG began with the ultimate moment of
subjective violence – the attempted annihilation of the human
species. The human cities – spread across twelve planets, or "twelve
colonies" – were destroyed with nuclear weaponry; a realization of
the paranoid, Cold War fantasy. The storyline of the first episodes
of BSG were focused on the destruction of the wealthiest human
city – *Caprica City*, on the *Caprica* colony. This annihilation was
depicted with pristine imagery of the glamorous city being reduced
to rubble in moments. In the first movie length episode – often
referred to as the mini-series since this was the style in which it
was initially aired – BSG delivered plenty of images reminiscent of
the 9/11 terrorist attacks and the ensuing "War on Terror" that has
seen the US military and the militaries of "willing" allies pursue
apparent terrorists to some distant corners of the globe. Viewers of
BSG witnessed the destruction of human civilization with blows
of spectacular violence. The depictions of the tumbling city-scapes

should be familiar to global witnesses of 9/11 and terrorism. These images show the viewer that remembering 9/11 is an important context for watching BSG.

I have identified two themes in BSG that I believe represent the most challenging side effects of the post-9/11 world. These themes are fear and racism. There are many other themes in BSG that would have been worthy of attention in this chapter (such as torture, military ethics, the role of the news media in reporting terrorism and war, and the links between democracy and fascism), but the two themes I have chosen are the most significant, the most powerfully represented in BSG, and the most relevant to the routine, mundane and everyday experience of living in the post-9/11 world. These themes are my way forward for analyzing subjective and objective violence in BSG and the "War on Terror".

Fear and Racism in the Human Fleet

Much has been documented of the post-9/11 political tactic of manipulating fears of terrorism or, perhaps more precisely, fears of another 9/11.[17] In their fearful responses to 9/11 some witnesses – whether they witnessed 9/11 via the news media or on the streets of New York City or Washington DC, or perhaps in a field in Pennsylvania – became "Stricken with fear and panic" and some "began to limit their travel … distrust others, and … surrender their freedoms willingly".[18] In many respects, this is not particular surprising. Terrorism is designed to spread fear and anxiety in a targeted audience. It is designed to have a lot of people watching, not just a lot of people dead.[19] Ott believes that BSG provides witnesses with some of the "symbolic resources" necessary to come to terms with the coordinates of the post-9/11 world through the deliberate evocation of the "Sept. 11 horrors".[20] In this way, the dramatization of terror themes in BSG – and other post-9/11 screen culture – provides a way of coming to terms with the horror of witnessing terrorism and of being a terrorists' target audience. As Ott argues:

> To understand the unique symbolic equipment that *BSG* affords for living in a post-9/11 world, it is vital first to establish the allegorical nature of the show. *BSG* begins with a surprise Cylon attack on the Twelve Colonies, which catches

the Colonial government and fleet flatfooted. Like the terrorist attacks of 9/11, the Cylon attack ... is organized by a
group of "monotheistic religious zealots" (read: Islamic fundamentalists) and executed with the aid of "sleeper agents
inside human society" (read: terrorists inside the U.S.).[21]

Ott adds that BSG provides viewers with a "vivid depiction" of
9/11 and helps witnesses understand a society at war. What is clear
in Ott's account is that the allegory of 9/11 in BSG represents something significant about the American capacity for symbolic equivalency and for fetishizing their disavowals.[22]

This capacity for symbolic equivalency and the associated
capacity for disavowal is well illustrated through the idea
seemingly adopted by several authors in the BSG studies canon that
fear of 9/11 somehow equates with fear of a human apocalypse.[23]
This equating should make most people cringe. This dilemma of
9/11's equivalency to other disasters sometimes plays itself out in
counterterrorism forums and conferences as well. I have had many
discussions with people who claim that 9/11 is the worst terrorist
attack of all time. I do not necessarily dispute such a claim, but I
often remind these people that in terms of casualties, destruction
and long-term potential for annihilation of a group of people 9/11
pales in comparison to the victimization of Jews by the Nazis before
and during World War II, the bombings of Hiroshima and Nagasaki,
atrocities in Northern Africa, and the decimation of East Timor to
name an horrendous few. Indeed, it should be considered a deep
insult (to the victims of all terror and war) to equate 9/11 with these
scandalous genocides. In symbolic terms however, this equivalence
relies on something other than a numbers game. Importantly,
9/11 was viewed live and direct from NYC and Washington DC.
In this way, it shares more with the initial scenes of devastation in
BSG than other more devastating acts of war or terror. BSG may
be a kind of symbolic manifestation of what was witnessed on
9/11 – this might be how some people in the US understood 9/11's
violence; *as a catastrophe, as a cataclysmic event, as an apocalypse.* I
must confess to also being prone to hyperbole on the night of 9/11.
I remember running to my parents' bedroom (I was 21 years old, an
undergraduate student, and lived in the family home at the time)

and declaring in my most dramatic prose that America was under attack, live on television; *do you want to see?* This exaggeration that witnesses like me were prone to on and after 9/11 points to a deeper malaise in terrorism and 9/11 research and theory: when terrorism occurs in the global south, the third world, and the underprivileged world it is viewed by Western governments, the media, policing organizations and academics as routine and a matter of course, but when it occurs in the global north, in wealthy metropoles such as New York, London and Madrid, the violence is treated as deeply abhorrent, as though all people must observe the sanctity of the violent act. This represents something close to what Žižek has described as "divine violence".[24] But in this instance, Žižek's description should be inverted, for it is not the divinity of the terrorists' violence that should be at stake, but the divinity of the supposedly holy and just reprisals that the US and its willing allies have carried out in 9/11's name. But here also lies the absurdity of the "War on Terror". Attacking the emotion *terror* with guns and bombs is something bordering on pathological.

9/11 sparked hyperbolic reactions in many witnesses. This reaction combined shock and horror with a certain compulsion to watch, even with a sick kind of excitement that was akin to rubber-necking at a car accident or stopping to capture a street fight with a mobile phone camera. This rubber-necking took on a global dimension courtesy of the global news media, and hyperbole was perhaps ensured. This is, at least partly, what Žižek was describing when he argued that 9/11 was "*jouissance* at its purest".[25] In a way, we *enjoyed* witnessing the destruction of a power that had reached an obscene level. On some unconscious level we enjoyed seeing the bully get their comeuppance. This idea is powerfully dramatized in the recent reality television program *Bully Beatdown* where bullies are identified and offered money to step into a ring with a professional fighter. Their resulting demise at the hands of a superior fighter is praised as a type of natural justice.[26]

This hyperbole should not, however, undermine the ability of BSG to shed light on some of the darker aspects of the response to 9/11. Among the post-9/11 fears that BSG reanimates is the fear of an enemy that looks like us, *an enemy that hides in plain sight*. As Melançon explains: "Shortly after the initial Cylon attack, the Fleet leadership learns that certain Cylon models look like humans. Five words are uttered in horror: 'They look like us now'".[27] The following dialogue is from episode two of season one. The dialogue is between two lovers, colonial fleet pilot "Boomer" and crew chief "Tyrol". Boomer discovers that several bombs have been removed from the amoury. She finds one in her duffel bag but she does not remember how it got there and she fears that it will be assumed that she is a Cylon sleeper agent if she reports it:

> *Boomer*: I took the one detonator from the duffel, replaced it, and then went back to my quarters.
>
> *Tyrol*: Well, ah … you know what? You know what? It's not your fault. Someone's obviously setting you up to take the fall for something, that's what it is. I mean, you wake up somewhere, you don't know how you got there or anything. You're drugged or manipulated. Or who knows what, something.
>
> *Boomer*: What do we do? 'Cause if I report what's happened, they're gonna think I'm a Cylon agent.
>
> *Tyrol*: No, they're not; no, they're not. No, no, no, why would they think that? That's crazy.
>
> *Boomer*: People are getting crazy, okay? You've heard the rumors: Cylons who look like humans, sleeper agents hiding in the fleet.[28]

There are three issues that I want to highlight from this dialogue. The first is that Boomer did turn out to be a sleeper agent, but she did not know it in this scene. Viewers later learn that it was part of her programming to awaken at designated times to unconsciously attempt acts of terror and espionage. She ultimately uses the bombs to tear open a section of *Galactica's* hull and releases most of the water supply into space. The second issue is that the fact she was a Cylon was not the security flaw in the human fleet that allowed Boomer to succeed in her unconscious plan. The security flaw rested in the fear and intolerance of the human fleet. The fact was that Boomer had lived and loved amongst humans, and this was where her conscious allegiances lay, even if her programming made her from time to time act out against this allegiance. Boomer wanted to report the missing bombs, but her fear of racial categorization and persecution prevented this. Lastly, much can be learned from Tyrol's response to her fears – *you're* not the Cylon agent. *You* have been set up. Someone else is the Cylon agent! For Tyrol a Cylon agent must exist (and he was right) but it must be someone other than his lover (on this point he was wrong).[29] Some hidden foreign agent must be to blame, but surely not someone I love and trust despite the evidence to the contrary!

Fears such as these could be witnessed throughout the human fleet despite no official acknowledgements from the government and the military that humanoid Cylons existed. Eventually however, Boomer's programming once again kicked in and she unconsciously attempted, but failed, to murder Commander Adama, the much-loved human military leader. Boomer was later murdered whilst in custody for this crime by Tyrol's flight-deck assistant, Cally. In a twist of fate (and of course, screen writing), Cally and Tyrol fell in love, married and had a child. When Tyrol also became aware that he was unconsciously a Cylon, he feared greatly for his relationship with Cally and their child. He was fairly certain that she would not understand that he was not an "evil" Cylon, but a "good" Cylon who loved humanity. Moreover, viewers come to learn that Tyrol, unlike Boomer, was not a dangerous sleeper agent waiting to be awakened to carry out acts of terror against the human fleet. He was, rather, one of the mysterious "final five" who wanted little more than peace with humanity. Tyrol's fears of being categorized and persecuted by Cally were realized in episode three of season four, "The Ties That Bind". In scenes from this episode viewers witness Cally learn that her husband is a Cylon and that their child, Nicky, is half-Cylon. Soon after learning this truth Cally encountered her husband in the quarters they shared:

> *Tyrol*: I know it's been a rough couple of weeks. I know what you're thinking. It's not true.
>
> *Cally*: It isn't?
>
> *[As he speaks, Cally sees flashbacks of their life together]*
>
> *Tyrol*: No. I'm not having an affair. I figured it out. I know

what's important. You're important. Nicky's important. We're important. Us. That's really what it's all about, isn't it? Family, a future. Building that future together. I promise you from now on I will be here for us. The three of us. Maybe the four of us. You know, maybe someday we, we'll have another baby. What do you think? Another baby? A brother, a sister for little Nick? What do you think, buddy? Hey? Would you like a little brother or sister?

[Cally, armed with a large wrench, beats Tyrol mercilessly, grabs Nicky, and leaves her husband for dead].[30]

Here we witness the problem at the heart of the Cylon dilemma. Through the terror that the humans experience, many become unable to fathom the idea of a "good" Cylon, a Cylon that might be their husband or wife, their son or daughter, their friends and family. Cally's terror becomes a metaphor for the dilemma of post-9/11 racism and discrimination. She is the embodiment of the inevitable and often nonsensical manifestations of post-terror fear. The objects of her fear (Cylons) were frozen into stability. Cally forced her love for her husband to be changed before allowing the object of her fear to be changed. When Cally learned that her husband and child were Cylons, she does not become aware that some Cylons are not monsters. She forced herself to become aware of something quite different – that she must change how she feels about her husband and child to accommodate her beliefs that every Cylon is a monster. This is something akin to a fundamental attribution error as it is sometimes called in psychological studies. When this error is made it is assumed that somebody exhibiting a particular, usually negative, trait is characterized by that trait. But if we were to ourselves exhibit that trait, we would not automatically assume that it was indicative of our character. In short, we assume the worst of others, but the best of ourselves. As such, Cally readjusted her perspective – instead of remembering all of those loving moments she spent with her family, she chose to re-remember – re-imagine – those moments and to re-interpret their meaning. These loving moments for Cally became part of a large-scale Cylon plot to annihilate humanity.

Cally's shifting perspective is not unlike the shift that occurred after 9/11 when racism and discrimination directed against people perceived to be Muslims became more frequent. Post-9/11 racism and discrimination may be viewed as a type of impotent acting out in search of the security that can be found in uniting against a universally feared and hated enemy. The Cylons play the rhetorical role of Muslims post-9/11. I do not mean to equate Muslims with a race of robots – I hope my words have not been taken on such a vulgar level. Rather I suggest that Muslims, like Cylons, are convenient scapegoats for other malaise within some societies. When the leadership of the Colonial Fleet finally discloses that there are Cylons that look human there was a predictable outcry: "Why were we not told" immediately?[31] The reason for this should be fairly clear in the post-9/11 world:

> The stated justification of the Fleet leadership for classifying the fact that some Cylons now look like humans is that they do not want to see neighbour turn against neighbour, create witch hunts, and see the social fabric ripped apart by paranoia … the Fleet must be protected *from itself.*[32]

This is a familiar tale. According to Freyd, anger directed at people perceived to be Muslim has been demonstrated on many occasions following 9/11.[33] A Lebanese man who had run the arts center at the World Trade Center was heckled as he was searching for survivors. A Wyoming mother and her children were chased from a "Wal-Mart" because they appeared Muslim. A mosque in Texas was fire-bombed. An Egyptian worker won a payout for discrimination after being fired from a restaurant because his manager believed that having someone who appeared Muslim as a staff member would be bad for business.[34] As I showed in chapter two, in research that I conducted in organizations in Melbourne, Australia I found that discrimination, racism and anti-Muslim sentiments had arisen as a result of 9/11 and the ongoing terror war. I could go on and on but my point is simple – 9/11 cleared a path for racism and discrimination to be directed against groups of people that are deemed to be responsible. This is also an account of repressive desublimation at work. In the face of trauma in NYC, its denizens found themselves in some instances unable to mediate their aggressive impulses. The aura of post-9/11 America meant that in some circumstances they were liberated to indulge in racist desires in a more socially permissible atmosphere. In this atmosphere the idea of a "good" Muslim became problematic for some people.[35]

A significant feature of post-terrorism discrimination and racism is the connections between language, aggression and violence. This is acknowledged in Ott's and Johnson-Lewis' analyses of BSG. As Ott argues, many despicable acts begin with the naming of the "Other" and the dehumanization that forges the Others' *Otherness*:

> if one does not see an enemy as human, then one does not feel compelled to treat "it" humanely ... The repeated references to Cylons as "machines", as well as the more derogatory use of the terms "toasters" and "skin jobs" function rhetorically to justify violence against all Cylons. In addition to degrading the Cylons, such language homogenizes them, reinforcing the prevailing perception that they are all the same and can thus be treated as one, nameless, faceless enemy.[36]

Ott argues that terms such as "extremists", "fundamentalists", "terrorists", and the "Axis of Evil" all perform a similar rhetorical role in the demonizing of Muslims after 9/11. The context of these words and phrases is George W. Bush's unfortunate post-9/11 declaration that you are either with us, or you are with the terrorists. Johnson-Lewis argues that Bush's words forge "terrorists" as an "undifferentiated mass" and that "It helps if terrorists are not actually people; it makes them much easier to kill".[37] I am sure what Johnson-Lewis means is "not actually people" like us; people in the same way that we are people. This de-humanization was again demonstrated by Cally. The following dialogue takes place immediately after she mercilessly beat her husband and fled with their child. She ran into a spacecraft launching bay pursued by another humanoid Cylon, Tory:

Tory: Cally!

Cally: Stay the frak away from me! I know what you are. I

know what all of you are. How could you?

Tory: We don't even know what we are.

Cally: I heard you. You're Cylons! A bunch of frakkin' skinjobs!

Tory: I wish it were that simple.

Cally, turning the key and closing the airlock behind Tory: I told you to stay away from me. Guess you better hope there's a spare body waiting for you!

Tory, holding her arms open wide: You want to kill me? Go ahead. Don't do this to yourself or to your child, to Nicky.

Cally: Get the frak away! You're not getting your hands on my son! Not you, not Galen [Tyrol]! He frakkin' used me!

Tory: He didn't know [he was a Cylon]! None of us did! We didn't find out until we entered that Nebula.

Cally: Oh, shut the frak up, traitor! Frak!

Tory: All we know is that we're Cylons. But in every other way, we're still the same people.

Cally: You're frakkin' machines!

Tory, looking at her hands: I don't know. But I do know that we're not evil. We're not inhuman. And we're just as scared and confused as you are.

Cally: I can't live like this! It's a frakkin' nightmare!

Tory, nearly weeping: You don't want to do this, Cally. He's your son![38]

Again, viewers witness Cally's racist attitudes at work as she considers whether she should kill herself and her child as a type of retribution against all Cylons. It is, in this sense, another example of repressive desublimation at work. Cally believed that Cylons had no right to live – for Cally, killing the Cylon sleeper agent, Boomer, was not killing at all. It was a legitimate act. This legitimacy was seemingly confirmed when Cally was charged for her crime and received only a few weeks imprisonment – as a member of the military her punishment for killing a colleague in ordinary circumstances would likely have been death. In the scene quoted above Cally was considering whether infanticide was also a legitimate course of action given the social and cultural contexts – the fact that her child was half human was seemingly irrelevant since Nicky was also half Cylon. Quite literally her hatred for Cylons outweighed her love of humanity. Her child's humanity was re-imagined as a non-humanity and she was willing to engage in suicidal violence if it meant ridding the world of another (half) Cylon. In the figure of Cally, we see the ultimate mindless racism – a racism that would see her condemn herself to death as punishment for her love of a Cylon. Cally's repressive desublimation is reminiscent of a skit performed by American comedian Dave Chappelle in which viewers see and hear the cautionary tale of a blind African-American man who was raised as a white supremacist. Upon learning that he is black he promptly leaves his wife because she is a "n**** lover".[39]

What is partially hidden amongst the accounts I have provided of outbursts of subjective violence in both BSG and the "War on Terror" – outbursts that have resulted in racial discrimination and fear of the Other – is the contours that sustain this violence. It is to these contours, or background, that I now turn.

The Background

For Žižek, objective violence is the symbolic and systemic violence that forms the background for spectacular and dramatic outbursts of subjective violence like terrorism, war and violent crime.[40] Analysis of violence in tele-visual culture has, perhaps for very good reasons, focused on representations of subjective violence and the subjective consequences of that violence for audiences of witnesses. Here I want to buck this trend and reflexively explore BSG with a focus on the backgrounded, objective and the visually benign systemic violence. If viewers of BSG were to focus on the background story they would witness Caprica City before it was destroyed – a decadent city characterized by ridiculous wealth, a wealth viewers come to learn is forged at the expense of cultural citizens that occupy working class roles, largely with multi-ethnic backgrounds.[41] The correlations with New York City should be obvious. NYC is a city of the elite and was the first target on 9/11. It is an epicenter for wealth and affluence, culture and hegemony. Much like Caprica

City, it is home to the affluent and worker, but also the poor, the unemployed, the drug addict, and the terrorist. Caprica City seems to have been modeled on New York City. Viewers of BSG are provided with many opportunities to admire Caprica City in the opening credits as the camera moves over the waters of a sun-kissed bay to capture a huge city littered with skyscrapers that seem to be erected directly on the coast line. The glamorous penthouse offices above, the sprawling masses below. One is struck by how reminiscent these scenes are of the morning of 9/11 – the sparkling sunlight and glistening water broken first by the city-scape on land, and then the smoke in the sky as it billowed from the Twin Towers. This similarity was also observed by Greene:

> the *Battlestar* series … never lets us forget the context of that devastation – the first shot in the credits every week is from the mini-series: an aerial shot flying into the Caprica skyline, much like the view that the terrorists would have had flying into lower Manhattan on 9/11. Whatever they may have meant before, after 9/11 images that simulate flying towards skyscrapers now connect us to that lonesome day.[42]

When Caprica City was reduced to rubble, the human denizens fled into space, a territory that they had no claim to. They were forced to shed their elite status and become members of the cultural underclass and what Georgio Agamben has described as *homo sacer* – people without a place or society, people who are not truly people.[43] It is homo sacer's place to toil and do little more than survive. With this shift the humans turned on each other and used violence whenever possible. On the fleeing human ships, societal structures re-established the comforting social norms of elitism and the underprivileged. Prostitution became common place and thugs and gangsters took control in some unpoliced segments of the fleet. This is the context in which we should also understand another enduring slogan from BSG – "All this has happened before, and all of it will happen again". The importance of this phrase in BSG has been explored by several authors in the *Battlestar Galactica Studies* canon.[44]

Casey, for example, points out that BSG has literally *happened* before. The original BSG "happened" in 1978 and was quickly followed by the rather lame *Galactica 1980* that deployed a storyline that is considered by some fans to be non-canonical.[45] It has since happened again in a post-9/11 world. In this world it has taken on different meanings, dimensions and consequences. But the phrase "All this has happened before, and all of it will happen again" has a far more important purpose in BSG. This purpose speaks to an inevitability that is inherent in the show's storyline and the storyline of the "War on Terror". It is an inevitability that does not fully play itself out until the re-imagined series concludes (sort of) after four seasons. This inevitability involves cycles of violence. These cycles of violence recreate past sins and past errors and ensure that the next moment of spectacular blowback is never far away.[46] The inevitability and predictability of these cycles of violence ensures that when violence and horror occurs it will repeat *the first time as a tragedy, but the second time as farce.*[47] This was the impetus behind the speech made by Commander Adama at the decommissioning ceremony for the Galactica shortly before the Cylons commence the human apocalypse. This speech is one of the first scenes in the re-imagined BSG:

> The cost of wearing the uniform can be high, but [long pause]. Sometimes it's too high. You know, when we fought the Cylons we did it to save ourselves from extinction. But we never answered the question 'Why?' Why are we as a people worth saving? We still commit murder because of greed, spite, jealousy. *And we still visit all of our sins upon our children.* We refuse to accept responsibility for anything we have done. Like we did with the Cylons. We decided to play God. Create life. When that life turned against us we comforted ourselves in the knowledge that it really wasn't our fault. Not really. You cannot play God then wash your hands of the things that you've created. Sooner or later the day comes when you can't hide from the things than you've done anymore.[48]

This is a particularly suggestive speech and one that has clear links to the post-9/11 world. Chomsky was quick to point out in the immediate aftermath of 9/11 that the hijackers and the architects were the products of training programs run by the Central Intelligence Agency (CIA) and other allied intelligence agencies in the 1980s.[49] The CIA is said to have played a significant role in "recruiting, training, and arming the most extreme Islamic fundamentalists it could find to fight a "Holy War" against the Russian invaders of Afghanistan".[50] The Afghan war against the Soviets fostered and hardened a fighting force from which it is generally believed that al-Qaeda emerged. This force then went looking for other fights and found them in Chechnya, Bosnia and Western China and later in Northern Africa, Washington DC and New York City. Chomsky argues that the CIA's support of Islamic fundamentalism was played down and in some cases totally denied after 9/11. Indeed, I have heard Bill O'Reilly suggest that no support was ever provided, accusing the son of a 9/11 victim of engaging in radical left-wing rhetoric when he suggested that the 9/11 hijackers were products of the US support of Islamic fundamentalism.[51] In fact, it is a matter of public record that the US government was still contributing funds to the Taliban regime throughout 2001 up until at least August 2 in part as reward for the "elimination of opium" cultivation in Afghanistan.[52] Yet, all one has to do is invoke pre-9/11 tele-visual culture to shed light on the American attitude towards the Afghan Mujahideen in the 1980s. Some are quick to forget that in the 1988 film *Rambo III* the US were depicted actively supporting Islamic fundamentalists in Afghanistan in their war against the Russian invaders. One impassioned speech by the American Colonel Trautman, Rambo's commander from a earlier film, reminds his Russian captors that the Mujahideen are "freedom fighters" who would "rather die than be slaves to an invading army. You can't defeat a people like that".[53] If only the US government had heeded Trautman's warning.

First as Tragedy ...

The debate over whether the US did or did not support Islamic extremism in the 1980s, a debate that could sometimes be heard on post-9/11 talk-back radio (in Australia and the US) and on some television news networks, misses the point. At that time, supporting the Mujahideen was likely the correct strategic decision. Surely we are sophisticated enough to know that 9/11 does not automatically mean that every decision made before 9/11 was simply in error? Regardless, the US support of Islamic fundamentalism in the 1980s is surely an example of *visiting all of our sins upon our children*. Stated differently 9/11 did not happen in an ahistorical vacuum. There were systematic and structural forces – a particular brand of US democracy, the fighting of a proxy war against the other Cold War superpower, a militarized everyday culture, Reganomics, a particular attitude towards the world, and a host of other objectively violent features – that formed the background for the subjectivity of US and Soviet led violence in many parts of the world. These conditions, along with many others, contributed to the hypersubjective violence that the world witnessed in real-time on 9/11. Or, as Žižek puts it, "while democracy can more or less eliminate constituted violence, it still has to rely continuously on constitutive violence".[54] The phrase *"All of this has happened before, and all of it will happen again"* becomes a little clearer. The violence currently being perpetrated by the US and its willing allies in the "War on Terror" may break up terrorist strong holds and places where terrorists move freely but the side-effect is that bombed foreign cities become the next breeding grounds and training camps for generations of terrorism to come. In short, fighting the war on terror – which has regularly involved fighting terror with terror – may do plenty to ensure that another 9/11 will occur.

Žižek believes that it is fear that keeps humanity grounded in perpetual repetitions of trauma and tragedy.[55] Žižek reminds us that "Twelve years prior to 9/11 … the Berlin Wall fell" and that this fall was supposed to usher in a new era of prosperity and human unity.[56] 9/11 has ushered in a new era of walls, but not only walls that are erected around large geographical regions. Rather, post-9/11 walls also surround gated communities and provide an illusory security to the planet's most wealthy inhabitants. Within these communities, a new class is emerging of people who "dine privately, shop privately, view art privately, everything is private, private, private".[57] But what links this new class is fear; *"fear of external social life itself"*.[58] Ironically, the acts of terror on 9/11 have imposed a terror from within, a terror that the wealthiest endure as a form of blowback for their affluence, as though they secretly agree with Ward Churchill's assessment of the wealthy professionals and business people who perished in the Twin Towers as "little Eichmanns".[59] These gated classes were perhaps equally "too busy braying, incessantly and self-importantly, into their cell phones, arranging power lunches and stock transactions, each of which translated, conveniently out of sight, mind and smelling distance, into the starved and rotting flesh of infants" as they hide out in the "sterile sanctuary" of the high-rises of the world's major cities.[60] This class distinction is most apparent for Žižek in São Paulo, Brazil – a city with "250 heliports" and some of the most dangerous city streets in the world.[61]

The farcical responses to 9/11 involved the erecting of walls wherever they would stand. These walls work to reinforce the inequality, hegemony and cultural domination that were the seeds of 9/11. The reproduction of this same inequality in Iraq and Afghanistan – or in the human fleet – will likely see history repeat. Whilst I cannot tell you where the next 9/11 will occur I can tell you that the next generation of terrorists will likely emerge in response to the protracted wars in Iraq and Afghanistan that have defined the first decade of the 21st century.

Conclusion: Should We Care About the Tyrant's Bloody Robes?

I want to conclude with something of a non-sequitur and a thought about *The Bourne Trilogy* films that star Matt Damon as a CIA trained killing machine, and how the films fit with what is at stake in this chapter.[62] The *Bourne* films tap into something dramatic about American culture. The stories of Jason Bourne depict a patriot, a man wanting only to make his beloved country safe and secure. But his desire is made impossible by the systemic conditions inherent in the US spy services, conditions that do little other than turn this patriot into an assassin who would kill anyone who does not share the CIA's limited worldview. For the leftist-liberal, these films represent moments of *jouissance* – moments of exhilarating enjoyment. Do you think the CIA does not wield this kind of power? Are you so naïve as to believe that this does not really happen? Of course it does. *It must* given the America that Jason Bourne serves.

The impact of these films is two-fold. First the viewer is reminded of the obscene subjective violence that the US wages around the globe in its theaters of the "War on Terror". Second, viewers are told to believe that there is a horrendous systemic, structural and objective violence that underpins this subjective violence and that this objective violence goes to the heart of what it means to be an American – *only a true patriot is willing to sacrifice what is needed*. Or, as the movies' crescendo reminds us, "Look at what they make you give". For the oppressed and the victims of US-led wars the propaganda is doubled. The subjective violence of US war efforts is combined with Hollywood depictions of objective violence (depicted in many other films such as *A Few Good Men, Enemy of the State*, and particularly the *X Files* television series and movies) to depict the US as the ultimate global evil. Can there be any doubt that would-be terrorists are being forged every day, some in the theaters of the US "war on terror", but perhaps also many others who are in the theaters of post-9/11 screen culture?

The re-imagined *Battlestar Galactica* seems designed to make the post-9/11 viewer consider when we should cry for the "tyrant's bloody robe".[63] This was the function of the post-9/11 cry, why do people hate America? But one does not need to hate America to understand the violent contours that made 9/11 possible. Indeed, the connections between the US funding and training of people who would later turn the gun on their trainers is fairly clear – and the US trained these people well in the tactics of terror. The 9/11 terrorists targeted sites of financial and military hegemony. The success of these attacks was *terror* at its purest. It is here that the suggestion of some canonical terror studies scholars that terrorism is random and arbitrary violence is revealed for its absurdity. The economic nerve-centre and the military brain are hardly random or incidental targets. Moreover, the plane that crashed in Pennsylvania was thought in some circles to be heading to the White House. The 9/11 attacks were far more precise than some of the US smart bombs deployed during post-9/11 wars.[64]

In both the short and long term it seems likely that fighting terror with terror is likely to create more terror. The recent attempt to detonate an underwear bomb on a flight between Amsterdam and Detroit is significant evidence of that. It is incredible that whilst fighting terror with bombs and guns in Afghanistan and Iraq is showing some results,[65] security staff at Western airports were not able to prevent an individual who was suspected of supporting radical ideologies from boarding an international flight with a bomb. More incredibly, this attempted attack has led to cries for profiling of potential terrorists (code for subjecting people who appear "Muslim" to greater scrutiny) – a further escalation of the systemic, objective violence; a violence that forms the contours of outbursts of subjective violence. Subjective and objective violence seem to feed on each other and the phrase "All of this has happened before, and all of it will happen again" is perhaps the best explanation of "progress" in the "War on Terror" – it is a progress towards repetition.

6.

Post-9/11 Comedy/Trauma

The secret courtesy that courses like ichor
Through the old form of the rude, full-scale joke.[1]

This chapter is divided into two parts. These parts are distinct but also deeply interconnected. They emerge from the same location and are therefore kin, yet, in some respects, seem to have little in common. The two parts to this chapter are drawn from post-9/11, tele-visual representations of *comedy* and *trauma*. To represent the distinction and interconnectedness of post-9/11 comedy and trauma I have adopted a strategy that is inspired by Julia Kristeva's work on mothering.[2] Whilst the subject matter of Kristeva's work is, of course, unrelated to the subject matter of this book, her method for representing disconnected yet intimately connected subjects seems ideal for my purposes here. As such, this is not only a chapter that is figuratively "in two parts" but rather, quite literally, cut in two. In the first half of this chapter I track a post-9/11 tele-visual culture of trauma using a variety of post-9/11 visual artifacts. I explore to this end the first post-9/11 monologues of David Letterman and John Stewart performing their routine and everyday roles as comedy talk show hosts. I also explore the "Sam Seaborn – Terror Expert" speech that was the centerpiece of a post-9/11 moment on *The West Wing*. These traumatic moments were sometimes glossed with comedy, a desire to both mourn and recover and, most importantly, a desire to return to *business as usual*. In the second half of this chapter I track a post-9/11 tele-visual culture of comedy. In this half of the chapter I focus on those moments when witnesses to post-9/11 tele-visual culture were encouraged to laugh – sometimes inappropriately and always uncomfortably – at the post-9/11 world and at 9/11's consequences. Rarely, if ever, was 9/11 directly laughed at. I show how trauma and comedy can be located side-by-side, as kin, in screen and tele-visual cultures in the aftermath of 9/11.

The chapter, like the others in this book, poses challenges of sifting through screen cultural "mess".[3] By sifting through this mess – and making judgments about what mess makes it into these pages, and which remain lying on the cutting-room floor in my tele-visual laboratory – I hope to progress further along in my account of what it means to witness terrorism, and what it means to talk about we in discussions about terrorism. This *"we"* has incorporated witnesses, locations and situations, and popular, tele-visual and screen cultural mediums for terrorism that have included television, film, and the blogosphere. In this chapter the witnesses are the viewers of some popular American television watching screens in locations throughout the world. I watched in Australia – a place that gives me a sense of distance but also an emotional connection to my fellow witnesses in the US and many other places where terrorism has occurred. In a way, this chapter is about their stories, but it is also about my own. It is also the stories of some hegemonic figures in American screen cultures. These figures have stories to tell, and their stories matter. The accounts of trauma in the first half of this chapter are drawn from television shows appearing shortly after 9/11. The weeks after 9/11 were a time for grief, a time for sorrow, and a time for coming to terms with the horror of what had happened. It should not be surprising that the accounts of trauma are littered with grief and sorrow, but also anger and rage. The accounts of comedy in the second half of this chapter take place, for the most part, several years after 9/11. Laughing at tragedy and horror is only possible once some time has passed. Laughing too soon would be deeply disrespectful to the victims of 9/11 and their families. Not laughing at all would perhaps award terrorists with the victory that they hoped for. In this way, laughing at the consequences of national tragedy might be a powerfully patriotic act; an act that represents recovery and catharsis. This is what I mean when I say that 9/11 itself was not really laughed at. It was the post-9/11 world, a world characterized by recovery and catharsis that is the butt of the joke.

Post-9/11 Trauma

In the first half of this chapter I do not intend to talk about trauma as a psychological or sociological concept, although this is part of the story. I have covered some of this ground already in chapter two where I explored the city as a "desert of the real"[4] and a "traumascape",[5] and in chapter four where I explored traumatic responses to 9/11 in *Friends*. Here, in the chapter's first half, I intend to continue pursuing post-9/11 trauma in tele-visual and pop-cultural locations. Of the many traumatic reactions to 9/11 that can be found in screen cultures, I have chosen three that I single out for special attention: David Letterman's monologue on *Late Show* that began the first post-9/11 episode; Sam Seaborn's question and answer session with students that were visiting the Whitehouse in post-9/11 *The West Wing*; and, John Stewart's monologue on *The Daily Show* that began the first post-9/11 episode. These accounts from a post-9/11 world are burdened with sorrow and grief, but also hope and defiance. The case of the character Sam Seeborn was also deeply condescending and is perhaps representative of a bubbling anger and resentment that some in the US held towards the world after 9/11. These three examples are drawn from important institutions in screen cultures. David Letterman and John Stewart are widely viewed on televisions from New York City to Melbourne and *The West Wing* was an exceedingly popular export to the world's screen cultural marketplace. As such, their contributions to post-9/11 tele-visual cultures hold special significance. Their contributions matter.

Letterman's Tribute: You Can Feel It, You Can See It

David Letterman's *Late Show*, holds a special place in tele-visual culture.[6] He has been a feature of late night television in many parts of the world since the 1980s and has occupied a central and sometimes political place on television.[7] When 9/11 occurred there was a sense that everything had changed. Very quickly this change was represented in television culture. Among the "first responders" to this cultural change, aside from the regular news media, were comedy talk shows such as Letterman's. As Letterman's show returned to air following 9/11 on 17 September 2001, he solemnly looked into the camera, shuffled in his seat, and began to talk:

> Welcome to the *Late Show*. This is our first show on the air since New York and Washington were attacked and I need to ask for your patience and indulgence here because I want to say a few things and believe me, sadly, I am not going to be saying anything new and in the past week others have said what I will be saying here tonight far more eloquently than I am equipped with to do. But if we are going to continue to do shows I just need to hear myself talk for a couple of minutes and so that is what I am going to do here. It is terribly sad here in New York City. We've lost 5000 fellow New Yorkers; and you can feel it. You can feel it, you can see it. It is terribly sad. Terribly, terribly sad. Watching all of this, I wasn't sure that I should be doing a television show because for 20 years we have been in the city making fun of everything, making fun of the city. Making fun of my hair, making fun of Paul [nervous laughter]. So to come to this circumstance that is so desperately sad, and I don't trust my judgment in matters like this.[8]

As I watched this monologue on one of the many available internet video media sites (in this instance, Google Videos), I transcribed what I heard and what I saw. Letterman was visibly shaken, but his voice did not break. But it was a solemn, post-disaster mood that confronted the viewer of the first post-9/11 episode of his iconic show. This is perhaps one of the more unique aspects of 9/11 as it sits in its place amongst a long history of major disasters – it was not only captured live and immediately analyzed, mined for meaning and replayed over and over again, but it occurred in the midst of a long-standing, tele-visual and pop-cultural history of New York City.

This is a central theme in the re-make of *The Day the Earth Stood Still*.[9] In the original film that was released in 1951, an alien diplomat lands in Washington DC – a logical place where the world's most powerful government and military is based and a location ideally suited for an alien/human diplomatic encounter. By 2008, Washington DC was no longer the most logical place for an alien diplomatic mission to land. A new and better location should be obvious to all – that location is Manhattan. If the goal is to reach the largest possible audience of witnesses and to address the world's leaders then surely Manhattan is the best place. The alien diplomat suggested that one of his driving influences was to land close to the United Nations building in Manhattan. But, the reasons must extend beyond this. Manhattan is among the world's most filmed locations and 9/11 was among the most filmed events in history. If alien races are observing this planet then they would surely know that cameras were already pointing at the Twin Towers when they were attacked and many more immediately after. Indeed, I was watching the attacks live in my house in the provincial city of Geelong in south-eastern Australia mere moments after the attacks began. The alien diplomats were undoubtedly hoping for the same real-time coverage. If these aliens had been watching Earth broadcasts, then they might have also noted the popularity of some television shows; *Friends, Sex and the City, Seinfeld, How I Met Your Mother, Spin City* to name a few. Manhattan was the natural setting for these shows, just as it would be for an alien race with a message to send.

David Letterman's is a familiar voice from Manhattan, a familiar voice from Ground Zero. This is why what Letterman has to say matters – Letterman's trauma matters. But, as Letterman explains, his was one voice among many. Some more important than others:

> But I will tell you the reason that I am doing the show and the reason that I am back to work is because of Mayor Giuliani. Very early on after the attack – and how strange does it sound to invoke that phrase, after the attack – Mayor Giuliani encouraged us and later implored us to go back to our lives, go on living, continue to try and make New York City the place that it should be.

Mayor Giuliani's position in American cultural life was renewed in the aftermath of 9/11. Letterman saw Giuliani as his motivator for returning to work, for returning to normal. 9/11 undermined and, in some instances, extinguished the everyday and banal routines of life; routines that structured time, existence and identity. Fromm argued that the routinization of everyday life, and the *"repression of the awareness of the basic problems of human existence"* that it allows, is of universal significance to human social life.[10]

> Man has to earn his daily bread, and this is always a more or less absorbing task. He has to take care of the many time- and energy-consuming tasks of daily life, and he is enmeshed in a certain routine necessary for the fulfillment of these tasks. He builds a social order, conventions, habits and ideas, which help him to perform what is necessary, and to live with his fellow man with a minimum of friction. It is characteristic of all culture that it builds a man-made, artificial world, superimposed on the natural world in which man lives.[11]

9/11 temporarily interrupted many of the banal yet psychically essential routines of day-to-day life. In some parts of Manhattan people stopped going to work, stopped shopping and lounging in coffee houses, stopped life. Not even television was exempt. The famous tele-visual phrase "we now return you to regular programming" was perhaps never as powerful as it was when television finally began returning to normal several days after 9/11. What is interesting about this aspect of post-9/11 television is that this experience was shared across the world by anyone who tuned in.

Right-wing commentator George Will believed that routines had helped sustain what he described immediately after 9/11 as America's "holiday from history".[12] Toby Miller and Ward Churchill have similarly argued that for the cosmopolitan inhabitants of Manhattan, everydayness involved a geographical and symbolic distance from global horrors.[13] But the "reality shattering" events of 9/11 showed us that not only was America not out of reach of the political violence and war that rages throughout the world, but that responding to this violence is, in itself, a reality shattering experience. As Žižek remarks of the immediate aftermath of 9/11[14]:

Now, we are forced to strike back, to deal with real enemies in the real world ... But *whom* to strike? Whatever the response, it will never hit the *correct* target, bringing us full satisfaction. The ridiculousness of America retaliating against Afghanistan cannot but strike the eye: if the so-called "only remaining superpower" destroys one of the world's poorest countries, in which peasants barely survive on barren hills, will this not be the ultimate case of an impotent passage *à l'acte*?[15]

The "impotent passage à l'acte" is a particularly noteworthy turn of phrase. "Passage à l'acte" is an expression capturing a type of acting out that is, depending on the context, sometimes associated with sexual encounters.[16] It is "impotent" because there was nothing in Afghanistan to reasonably destroy. When Žižek questions whether the "ultimate irony" of the invasion of Afghanistan shortly after 9/11 is that its capital Kabul "already looks like downtown Manhattan after 11 September", is he not essentially asking the question; *How can America fuck something that is already fucked*? Perhaps this is the best context to understand the "DON'T FUCK WITH US, WE FUCK BACK" bumper stickers that I discussed in an earlier chapter.

The invasion of Afghanistan became politically, ideologically and socially possible in the days following 9/11.[17] One of Letterman's guests on the first post-9/11 show was news anchorman Dan Rather. Rather fought back tears throughout his time on the program. He had played a central role in disseminating 9/11 in real-time to witnesses throughout the world and it seemed that it had taken a toll. I was moved by Rather's words at times and I felt a deep sorrow for everybody who had been devastated by the attacks. But I was also aware that many of Rather's words sat uneasily with me. He was barely concealing his rage and his desire for revenge. He called for the US government to "turn out the lights all over Afghanistan" and he believed that "they [the US government/ military] could have turned off all communication; why they didn't do that we'll have to see later".[18] I can think of at least one reason that the US government did not "turn out the lights", at least initially – it may have led to the unnecessary deaths of innocent people in Afghanistan in the confusion that such an action would cause. What did Rather even mean by "turning out the lights"? I am tempted to suggest that Rather believed that the CIA or the US military are in possession of some kind of doomsday device that knocks out power systems (it is not inconceivable that such capability probably exists). Perhaps Rather was referring to a bombing campaign that would target critical power infrastructure. Ironically, it is believed by some counterterrorism practitioners and academics that Western cities are vulnerable to terrorists similarly targeting such power infrastructure. Regardless of the specific meaning(s) that Rather intended, it seems clear that he desired a swift retribution attack against an ill-defined enemy, in this case Afghani civilians.

Later in this interview, Rather began to occupy a position that is something akin to a "Dr Phil" of counterterrorism. He presumed to diagnose what is wrong with "terrorists":

Rather: they hate America, they hate us, it isn't that they – this is one thing that makes this war different they don't want territory, they don't want what we got, they want to kill us and destroy us, it's a, you know, it's a heavy statement but it's true, they seek to accomplish our death, our death as a people, as a society and a culture … they see themselves as the world's losers, they would never admit that, they see us, we have everything, we win everything, this is their view of things, they see themselves as, you know, we should be a great people but we're not, and it drives them batty, that's the only explanation.

Letterman: Envy? It's just envy, jealousy, bitterness?

Rather: Deep abiding hate, which – *it's very difficult for anyone in western civilization much less our United States of America to understand this kind of hate,* you have to see it first hand, you have to of been among it to understand it's, it – there's no rationality to it by *our standards,* there's no trying to explain it, but I keep coming back to the point. David, it's a mistake to believe this has anything to do with the Islamic religion, these are crazy people, they are haters, they hate us for who and what we are, they don't want anything except to see us dead and see us destroyed.[19]

Rather might be seen here to be tapping into what Miller describes as the "mythic folksiness" of 9/11.[20] This folksiness has framed America as a nation only capable of good and righteousness. Views such as Rather's, transmitted to Letterman's audiences throughout the world, did not paint America in a positive light. Views like these did little to quell the emerging anti-Americanism that was spreading quickly as US war-making was mobilized. Sardar and Davies argue that a moment of "universal sympathy" for America quickly transformed into "a growing fissure" in attitudes towards America.[21] It is a fissure to which comments like Rather's can only have contributed.

It is particularly noteworthy that Sardar and Davies' two books on American culture begin with chapters on the meanings and consequences of 9/11.[22] These attacks and the central role they play in American and global societies have provided a space in which some powerful myths have emerged. As Sardar and Davies argue:

> In America the footprints of history have been overlaid by the creation of mythic narratives that convey the idea of America. How America thinks about its place in the world is a direct expression of its idea of national mission, a story explained by its mythic tradition which has determined how its cultural and strategic history has advanced since 9-11.[23]

Rather was engaging with this mythic narrative when he suggested that it must be hard for people in the US to imagine the kind of hate that the 19 hijackers must have felt and that "our standards" would not allow for this kind of violence. But I am not suggesting that Dan Rather is anything other than a man in grief, and grief can lead to all manner of acting out in frustration and impotent rage. I cannot imagine taking the role that Rather played during 9/11 as a disseminator of horrific violence; I probably could not have done it. But Rather's comments on Letterman make me feel uneasy because Rather is somebody important – Rather's trauma matters, and his impotent rage has consequences.

Sam Seaborn's Rant: Learning Terrorism from the Ignorant

9/11 myth-making was also demonstrated in a post-9/11 episode of *The West Wing*.[24] Audiences witnessed in this episode the character Sam Seaborn make a righteous speech about terrorism – an area in which Sam Seaborn "dabble[s]"[25] – to a group of school children. I have probably never been as offended as someone who studies terrorism as I was by this clip from *The West Wing*. His lack of knowledge and the pompous certainty with which he delivered the message was cringe-worthy. The fact that Seaborn is a fictional character is cold comfort. Poniewozik has similarly picked up on this in an article for *Time* magazine. He argues that this "Terrorism 101" episode whilst "earnest in its tone" was "God-awful in its condescending pedantry" that "rachet[ed] up the show's already problematic preachiness to levels you couldn't reach with a 50-foot pulpit".[26] Perhaps most alarming about Seaborn's glib account of terrorism was that it was delivered to school children in a quasi-classroom setting, ringing metaphorical bells indicating that the children of the world were about to hear some truth-bombs.

> *Student*: You know a lot about terrorism?
>
> *Sam Seaborn*: I dabble
>
> *Student*: What are you struck by most?
>
> *Sam Seaborn*: There's a 100% failure rate.
>
> *Student*: Really?
>
> *Sam Seaborn*: Not only do terrorists always fail at what they are after, they pretty much always succeed in strengthening whatever it is they are against.
>
> *Student*: What about the IRA?
>
> *Sam Seaborn*: The Brits are still there. The process is still there. The Basque terrorists have been staging terrorist attacks in Spain for decades with no result. Left wing Red Brigades from the 60s and 70s, the Baader-Meinhoff Gang in Germany to the Weathermen in the US have tried to overthrow capitalism. You tell me. How is capitalism doing?

The inflated motives ascribed to terrorists' causes allows the myth of the "unsuccessful terrorist" to flourish. To suggest that the IRA and anti-capitalist terror groups "always fail" is to misunderstand the power of terrorism to generate fear, terror and anxiety in witnesses in places both near and distant to terrorism's flashpoint. Whilst the IRA did not rid all of Ireland of the British, it is hard to dispute that they achieved many goals that include political legitimacy, widespread sympathy and support from diasporic and non-diasporic communities in many diverse parts of the world, as well as some strategic gains. Moreover, if publicity is the oxygen of terrorism then the IRA breathed easily.[27] Their popularity is testament to the success of spectacular violence in generating audiences of witnesses.[28] The IRA may have wanted the British out, but this alone cannot determine whether they succeeded or failed. The same can be argued for a host of left-wing terrorist groups from the 1960s-1980s. Certainly capitalism was not overthrown in the Western Democratic nations where they concentrated at least some of their violence, but they still killed, maimed and attracted enormous amounts of publicity and spread terror, fear and anxiety. But Sam Seaborn was not done:

Student: But weren't we terrorists at the Boston Tea Party?

Sam: Nobody got hurt at the Boston Tea Party. The only people that got hurt were the fancy boys who didn't have anything to wash down their crumpets with. Jumped out from behind bushes while the British came down the road in their bright red jackets, but never has a war been so courteously declared. Parchment and calligraphy. Your highness we beseech on this day in Philadelphia to bite me if you please.

Attitudes such as these are nothing new as Noam Chomsky has spent large parts of his career arguing; it is *our enemies'* crimes that are terrorism, not *ours*.[29]

Student: Well what do you call a society that has to just live everyday with the idea that the pizza place you're eating in could just blow up without any warning?

Sam: Israel

This is a fairly lame answer to a legitimate question from one of the students. Seaborn had an opportunity to slightly redeem his indulgent speech by answering "a democracy" but he instead chose to play to the political temperament of the conservative world and answer "Israel". I am not suggesting that Israelis are not subjected to a long running terrorist threat, but I would like to suggest that Israel is not a reasonable substitute or synonym for the only obvious ending to Sam's speech which was "a democracy". This answer would have included the struggle of all democratic nations against terrorism, not just Israel's.

Seaborn's rant put the world in its place. It informed those who had concerns about terrorism and the US's own history of violence that they were naïve and that their doubts were unfounded. It also served as a reminder that *we* were the *illegitimate* targets of terrorism and we should be humanized in the same breath that our enemies should be demonized. The school children take the place of hopeless, dim-witted nation states that naively protect terrorists and further the cause of terrorism through not fully supporting American ideals.

But what I have learnt in the years that I have studied American 9/11 culture is that many American's are as frustrated as I am by US anti-terror cheerleading. Chief among these cultural critics is John Stewart. His post-9/11 tribute to the 9/11 victims and New York City – his home – showed the world a glimpse of why we should have sympathy for the trauma that American's suffered on 9/11. Understanding John Stewart's tribute might go a long way to mending the negative perceptions of America and Americans that exist in some parts of the world.

John Stewart – "Are you okay?"

There is a humility about John Stewart; a quality rarely found in television personalities. This humility is combined with a quick wit, high intelligence, and a knack for comedic phrasing. John Stewart is an important figure in the "soft news" category of American journalism.[30] Stewart regularly plays host to presidential hopefuls, renowned authors, academics, sports personalities, politicians and entertainment celebrities. It is believed that young people make up a significant proportion of his viewing audience.[31] This at one point prompted *Fox News* pundit Bill O'Reilly to describe John Stewart's audience as comprised of 87% "stoned slackers".[32] This is how John Stewart began his first post-9/11 episode:

> Good evening and welcome to *The Daily Show*. We are back. This is our first show since the tragedy in New York City. There is no other way to start this show than to ask you at home the question that we asked the audience here tonight and that we've asked everybody that we know here in New York since September 11 and that is, are you okay? And we pray that you are and that your family is. I am sorry to do this to you. It's another entertainment show beginning with an overwrought speech of a shaken host and television is nothing if not redundant. So, I apologise for that. It's something that, unfortunately, we do for ourselves so that we can drain whatever apses that is in our hearts and move on to the business of making you laugh. Which we haven't been able to do very effectively lately. And everyone has checked in already. I know we are late. I'm sure we are getting in right under the wire before the cast of Survivor offers their insight into what to do in these situations [nervous laughter]. They said to get back to work and there were no jobs available for a man in the foetal position under his desk crying [laughter]. Which I gladly would have taken [laughter]. So I come back here.[33]

For Stewart, his post-9/11 address was not a moment for anger, impotent rage or prejudicial hatred – things that would quickly turn sympathy into disgust. Stewart just wanted to know if we, the viewers, were "okay". With this address we also witnessed a common theme amongst many people with post-9/11 tele-visual air-time; the call to return to what we were doing before 9/11, to return to our everyday routines and habits, to get back to business as usual. In this way John Stewart was echoing other figures like David Letterman and Rudy Giuliani. It is hard to dispute that 9/11 had a decisively de-routinizing effect. As Fromkin once suggested, terrorism befuddles the mind and paralyses the will to resist living with the constant fear and anxiety of further terrorism.[34]

In a post-9/11 world Ulrich Beck and Elizabeth Beck-Gernsheim argue that "certainties have fragmented into questions which are now spinning around in people's heads".[35] 9/11 introduced many uncertainties to the everydayness of city living. Moments that were taken for granted such as the commute to work on public transport, residing or working in the highest reaches of a city's skyscrapers, and congregating in one of the many public spaces that the city offers have lost their charm. They no longer offer the assurances of safety that they once seemed to promise. Since "Social action needs routines in which to be enacted", and where "our thoughts and actions are shaped, at the deepest level, by something of which we are hardly or not at all aware", the 9/11 attacks, and the devastating acts of terrorism that have occurred before and since, have struck at the heart of city-living.[36] This is what I was referring to when I described the city as the terrorists' playground: "a place where the most physical, psychological and emotional damage can be inflicted".[37]

A New American Dream

Many post-9/11 tele-visual moments give viewers reasons to mourn for America. These reasons do not have to be accompanied by forgetfulness of the US's vicious and murderous post-9/11 retributions. Nor do they have to lead to the glorification and deification of the American way of life. I think it is enough to hear stories and allow ourselves to feel sad and to remember. This is how John Stewart concluded his first post-9/11 monologue:

> The main reason that I wanted to speak tonight is not to tell you what this show is going to be, not to tell you about all the incredibly brave people that are here in New York and in Washington and around the country. But we've had an unenduring pain here, an unendurable pain and I wanted to tell you why I grieve [voice breaking] but why I don't

despair. I'm sorry [quietly]. Luckily we can edit this [laughter]. One of my first memories is of Martin Luther King being shot. I was five. And if you wondered if this feeling would pass. When I was 5 and he was shot, here's what I remember about it. I was in a school in Trenton. And they shut the lights off and we got to sit under our desks. And we thought that was really cool. And they gave us cottage cheese. Which was a cold lunch because there was rioting but we didn't know that, we just thought "My God, we get to sit under our desks and eat cottage cheese". And that's what I remember about it. And that was a tremendous test of this country's fabric and this country has had many tests before that and after that. The reason I don't despair is because this attack happened. It's not a dream. But the aftermath of it, the recovery, is a dream realized. [voice breaking] And that is Martin Luther King's dream. Whatever barriers we've put up are gone. Even if it is just momentary. And we're judging people by not the color of their skin, but the content of their character. All this talk about these guys are criminal masterminds. They've got together and they've, their extraordinary guile and their wit and their skill. It's a lie. Any fool can blow something up. Any fool can destroy. But to see these guys, these firefighters, these policemen, and people from all over the country, literally with buckets, rebuilding. That's extraordinary. And that's why we've already won. It's light. It's democracy. We've already won. They can't shut that down. They live in chaos. And chaos, it can't sustain itself. It never could. It's too easy and it's too unsatisfying. The view from my apartment [voice breaking] was the World Trade Center [long pause]. And now its gone. And they attacked it. This symbol of American ingenuity, and strength, and labor, and imagination and commerce, and it is gone. But you know what the view is now? The Statue of Liberty. The view from the south of Manhattan is now the Statue of Liberty. You can't beat that.

This statement could be analyzed, deconstructed, attacked for its inaccuracies (ask an American Muslim or an African-American if people were judged by the color of their skin after 9/11), but I am going to choose a different path, a path that allows me to draw the first half of the chapter to a close. This closure is a point at which we must take care in how we choose to remember, and perhaps even pay tribute, to those who were killed or who continue to suffer as a consequence of 9/11. As Žižek highlights:

> Why should the World Trade Center catastrophe be in any way privileged over, say, the mass slaughter of Hutus by Tutsis in Rwanda in 1994? Or the mass bombing and gas-poising of Kurds in the north of Iraq in the early 1990s? Or the Indonesian forces' mass killings in East Timor? Or … the list of countries where the mass suffering was and is comparably greater than the suffering in New York, but which do not have the luck to be elevated by the media into the sublime victim of Absolute Evil.[38]

In a sense, 9/11 has received so much attention because so many images were witnessed. History is far more palatable when it can be seen by an audience first-hand, whether in reality or *hyperreality*.[39] But, we should remember that in terms of loss of life and in terms of ability and resources at hand to rebuild and recover, the US will survive in prosperity and affluence. In many respects, the US military response to 9/11 has been far more devastating in terms of death and destruction. The US has, mostly, bounced back from 9/11 whilst Afghanistan and Iraq continues to suffer. World history has shown that "insane fanatics" cause a lot less damage than "rational strategists"[40] – "There is much more ethical insanity in a military strategist planning and executing large-scale bombing operations than in an individual blowing himself up in the process of attacking the enemy".[41]

Post-9/11 Comedy

When academic Giselinde Kuipers arrived in the US on 12 September 2002, the day after the first anniversary of 9/11, she was told that "September 11 was the death of comedy" and that 9/11 marked the beginning of a time when "Americans have stopped laughing".[42] Kuipers notes that one year after 9/11 "Humour *about* 9/11" was certainly not funny. It was not funny for Chandler to make a joke about a bomb in an airport in a post-9/11 episode of *Friends*; so the storyline was changed and the episode was re-shot.[43] It was no longer funny for Homer to be pitted against New York City in a 1997 episode of *The Simpsons*; so there was hesitation from major networks when it came to re-airing this episode of the über-popular and syndicated show.[44] In the second half of this chapter I do not intend to talk about comedy as a psychological and sociological concept, although this is part of the story. Post-9/11 screen and tele-visual culture has offered plenty of opportunities to laugh again, and sometimes laugh at the post-9/11 world (but rarely at 9/11 itself). From *The Simpsons* to *Family Guy* and *American Dad*, to *Team America: World Police*, the second half of this chapter shows how the world is learning to laugh at the post-9/11 world. But how should we interpret this laughter? Does it show that America and the world has recovered, or are at least beginning to recovery? Or, are these moments of post-9/11 comedy insults of the highest order? Funny or demeaning? A roast or an insult?

9/11 jokes should be viewed as something akin to a "roast". When conducted delicately, roasts can be a rite of passage, a cathartic moment, and a sign of transition. Yet, roasts can also be "taken too far" and can quickly become disrespectful, deeply offensive and spectacularly insulting. I explore some of these roasts here. I focus my attention on some popular cartoons; *The Simpsons*, *Family Guy*, and *American Dad*. I also explore the plucky puppets in the film *Team America – World Police*. I have chosen these programs because they occupy important pop-cultural, tele-visual and post-9/11 spaces both in the US and throughout the world. They offer a partial view of the post-9/11 world and their popularity is evidence of a culture of witnessing in post-9/11 popular, tele-visual and screen cultures.

They Stick All of the Jerks in Tower One

In the audio commentary that is part of the array of special features in the season nine DVDs of *The Simpsons*, one particular episode's commentary stands out from the rest. It is the audio commentary that accompanies episode one of season nine; "The City of New York vs. Homer Simpson".[45] In this 1997 episode, Homer's friend

Barney takes Homer's car around America on an alcohol-fuelled bender. After being missing for several months, Barney suddenly reappears and Homer discovers his car has been abandoned in New York City. Homer arranges to visit New York and retrieve his car despite revelations of his long-standing vow to never return to NYC after he was repeatedly mugged on his first trip there. Homer arrives to discover that his car is parked between Tower One and Tower Two.[46] From Homer's arrival at the World Trade Center the episode is set at the iconic location – sometimes waiting in the plaza between the Towers for parking inspector Steve Grabowski who can remove the wheel clamp that prevents Homer from moving his car, other times searching for the bathroom in both Towers and conversing with the Towers' inhabitants (that is, people who are supposedly living in the Towers in this fictional NYC).

In the DVD audio commentary, three of this episode's creators discussed the cartoon images of the World Trade Center that they had produced and their meaning in a post-9/11 world.

> *Bill Oakley*: The elephant in the room with this episode as most of you who originally saw it may know is that it is all primarily about the World Trade Center. So, a sensitive topic and I understand that it has been pulled from syndication and it actually hasn't aired for any at all since September 2001.
>
> *Josh Weinstein*: Is that true? I thought that they had finally started to put it back into rotation.
>
> …
>
> *Bill Oakley*: I was always a big fan of the World Trade Center. I went there when they finished, when they finished it when I was six or seven years old. Every time I went to New York pretty much I would go to the top and I did it shortly before we did this episode. And then we sent Silverman actually because one of the things we wanted to do was make this a fairly realistic although Simpsonized depiction of the streets of New York. So Dave Silverman went with a camera, took hundreds and hundreds of photos of the area around the World Trade Center and all the buildings and the pizza par-

lors and even like the cones they use, the traffic cones.

Josh Weinstein: Right, and I even recognize the other buildings that were destroyed.

Bill Oakley: Oh right, the other buildings that were destroyed can be seen in this episode.

Jim Reardon: I think September 11th happened, I know that beyond what it did to everybody in the studio, the guys that designed that stuff had an extra feeling of pain. This was the stuff that they had drawn that was no longer there.

Bill Oakley: It's very odd and I know that things like even the awnings of the pizza place across the street were carefully color matched and so forth ... normally in *The Simpsons* it's not the most realistic ... but this one was. And even like the observation deck and the elevator and stuff all looks exactly like it did at the World Trade Center so it's rather eerie to see it today.[47]

It is in this context that the World Trade Center can be seen to embody what some social theorists and psychoanalysts might call the "thing". Kay describes the "thing" as that "seemingly humdrum object" that acts as a banal structural component of everyday life that has the capacity to burst forth and "disclose its cosmic relevance".[48] Martin Heidegger's concept of the "thing" is particularly noteworthy for my purposes here.[49] For Heidegger, we describe something as a "thing" if it is near, has use, and if it is something that must first be reachable as a concept before it can be reachable as an object. If we can imagine something's use, or something's value, then it might be said to have a "thingly" quality.[50] Heidegger's essay on the "thing" is framed in the context of an explosion of communications technologies that were shrinking time and space and where the abolition of distance found its apex in television which, according to Heidegger, would "soon pervade and dominate the whole machinery of communication".[51] The "thing" can fade into the background in one instance, but in another instance the witness cannot look away. In one sense, it can be distant. Through television it is also somehow in our living rooms. What the discussion between the episode's creators shows is that the Twin Towers were "things" of "cosmic relevance" long before 9/11. Baudrillard[52] and Žižek referred to the power of the Twin Towers as the "thing" when they argued that the terrorists carried out the attacks, but we wished for it,[53] *we* wished for the ultimate special "effect", the ultimate destruction of obscene power.[54] Baudrillard, in turn, described this as the "terroristic imagination which dwells in all of us".[55]

> The fact that we have dreamt of this event, that everyone without exception has dreamt of this event – because no one can avoid dreaming of the destruction of any power that has become hegemonic to this degree – is unacceptable to the Western moral conscience. Yet it is a fact, and one which can indeed be measured by the emotive violence of all that has been said and written in the effort to dispel it.[56]

The Twin Towers were already "things" before 9/11 (symbols of hegemonic power, cultural and financial oppression and also commercial achievement, engineering mastery and ingenuity), and unmistakeably "things" in a post-9/11 world (targets of international terrorism and war, a site for blowback; perhaps even taking over from Coca-Cola as the real thing!). The Towers can be seen in many pre-9/11 images of the New York City skyline. They were objects in one sense; they were real, they were situated in lower Manhattan. But, they were reachable as a concept – as a symbol of American economic prowess, a prowess that was undermined on 9/11. They were a symbol of American hegemony, a site for unbridled profiteering and possibly even the "technocratic corps" at the heart of America's corporate-military complex.[57] The Towers had even been targeted before; in 1993 by a group that was suspected to have links to a Saudi "billionaire"[58] in the days when Osama bin Laden was not a household name. Perhaps Baudrillard and Žižek were right – we knew that 9/11 was possible, or perhaps even inevitable, as a kind of blowback of corporate America's perceived greed, a greed that was on show during the early days of the global financial crisis. Have we not all longed for the bully to get his comeuppance? Or, in my more psychoanalytic moments, does not every beaten boy look forward towards destroying the abusive father's brute force, idiotic rage and power?[59]

The Twin Towers as the "thing" reaches its crescendo in a joke in this episode of *The Simpsons*, a joke that executive producer Bill Oakley describes as "regrettable" and "cringe-worthy"[60]—"they stick all the jerks in Tower One".[61] As a result of this joke already existing when 9/11 occurred, it was decided that it had to be removed. As Josh Weinstein observed, "some of the jokes have extra heavy meanings [after 9/11], of course they had no meanings [before 9/11]".[62] This episode of *The Simpsons* – a marquee episode that begins season nine – was pulled from syndication as part of a post-9/11 fetishistic disavowal (as described in chapter four). Given that this episode can still be found on the season nine DVD complete with audio commentary and has since returned to syndication, this disavowal was an impotent gesture that was unable to delay the inevitable confrontation between witnesses, the missing buildings and the hole in the ground at Ground Zero in the cartooned world of *The Simpsons*.

Perhaps because of this, *The Simpsons* were slow to find the post-9/11 world funny. For a program that has long occupied a subversive place in prime-time television, regularly engaging in cynical political commentary and criticism of the media, *The Simpsons* was mostly, and oddly, quiet on terrorism and 9/11 in its post-9/11 episodes.[63] One was far more likely to find a dig at *Fox News* than a 9/11 reference. I have nonetheless identified some important moments when *The Simpsons* played a central role in laughing at the post-9/11 world. Two post-9/11 episodes in particular stand as a testament to returning laughter in a program that was slow to find this new world funny.

In episode six of season sixteen Homer, Apu, Ned Flanders and Grandpa Simpson cross the border into Canada to purchase prescription medications that they are unable to get in the US (making many jokes about the ease with which drugs can be obtained in Canada along the way).[64] As they try to cross the border back into the US, an unfortunate set of circumstances creates the impression that Apu is a would-be terrorist determined to carry out an attack on US soil. Apu takes a sip of extremely hot coffee that makes him shriek in a style befitting a suicide bomber that is about to detonate his bomb-vest (aye yai yai yai yai yai yai! – at least this is what the cultural stereotype of the suicide bomber would lead us to believe). Seeing his friend in pain, Ned raps a wet towel around his head to cool him down just as Homer's car pulls up to the checkpoint to enter the US from Canada. The image of the Islamic fundamentalist suicide bomber is complete. *The Simpsons* effortlessly tapped into the anxieties of the post-9/11 world in what was their first serious attempt to represent 9/11's meanings and consequences. This same theme was the subject of a season twenty episode[65] that was praised by the *Council on American-Islamic Relations* for its "challenging" of Muslim stereotypes.[66] In this episode, Bart befriends a Muslim boy who is subjected to discrimination and racism by the usual bullies at Springfield Elementary (Kearney, Dolph and Jimbo). His name is "Bashir" prompting Dolph to remark that he "love[s] a kid that comes with directions" (*bash-here*).[67] Bart engages with the multicultural delights of tasting exotic foods and dancing exotic dances. Homer comes to believe that Bashir's father is plotting to blow up the Springfield Mall. Homer is right in a way. He is planning to blow up the mall, but not as a terrorist, rather as an engineer employed to carry out a controlled destruction to make way for the new Springfield Mall. Homer quickly realizes, in a way that only Homer can, that he has been a bigoted fool, and makes an effort to also appreciate the multicultural delights that can be found in the Muslim Other.

This episode was praised for depicting negative Muslim stereotypes as idiotic and absurd and worthy of the ridicule that *The Simpsons* sling. In a letter to Matt Groening, Hussam Ayloush, Executive Director of the *Council on American-Islamic Relations*, wrote that the episode:

> By introducing a professional Muslim family … highlighted the diverse make-up of Springfield and brought to light how Americans can work toward mutual respect and inclusion by getting to know their neighbors. The episode also builds on the values that have made America the great nation that it is – a nation in which citizenship is about finding common ground and building a better society. American Muslims have been doing just that by making daily con-

tributions to our society that often go unrecognized. I hope you will continue to use humor to help all Americans see other perspectives on important social issues.[68]

But, as always, who is watching matters, and what I have described as a *sociology of we* in the first chapter is revealed once again to be a complex construct. In response to the same episode, a spokesperson for Britain's "The Islamic Cultural Centre + The London Central Mosque" hoped that "Muslims take no notice of the show". This episode was viewed by some to be disrespectful, particularly Homer's reference to Allah as "Oliver" and to The Koran as "The Corona".[69]

It would seem that *The Simpsons* has played a prominent role in post-9/11 popular, tele-visual and screen cultures despite, for the most part, the show's creators finding 9/11 and the post-9/11 world unfunny. But, even if 9/11 is not funny and if we believe that there is no role for cathartic humor in the face of disaster, might we still cling at least to the sense of irony and the humor that it promises? Might 9/11 provide a space for such an irony, an irony that allows us to laugh at 9/11's meanings and consequences, without laughing at 9/11? Is there more catharsis to be found in post-9/11 irony?

Post-9/11 Irony

Roger Rosenblatt's[70] assessment of what had changed after 9/11 was fairly simple; "this [9/11] will mark the end of the age of irony". For Rosenblatt, in the years before 9/11, Americans – "we" in Rosenblatt's words – had been lulled into a type of complacency and a belief that the world's distant problems would remain distant:

> For 30 years, just about as long as the twin towers were up, we have been operating under an attitude that things were not to be believed in, that nothing was quite to be taken seriously and that nothing was real. Nothing could have been more real than the savage zealots who hit the twin towers and the Pentagon and who caused the plane to go down in Pennsylvania. So one change certainly will be that the smirk on American intelligent life, the idea of giggling and thinking that nothing was serious, that's certainly going to change.[71]

I hope to show in this section that irony is alive and well. More than this; 9/11 has sparked its own ironic turn that takes shape in some well-known post-9/11 comedy television. But before I confront some of this tele-visual culture head-on, I must first outline a way to understand post-9/11 irony.

For sociologist Bryan Turner, post-9/11 irony is closely linked to patriotism.[72] Turner believes that "[c]osmopolitan virtues" require a certain "methodological irony". In what might be described as an age where multicultural harmony has become strained, and in the midst of some well known but rather odd declarations of a supposed "clash of civilisation"[73], the acceptance of multicultural and cosmopolitan city living requires an "ironic or disinterested distance" from one's own culture.[74] Yet, perhaps paradoxically, Turner also argues that this ironic distance can only be possible "once one already has an emotional connection to a place".[75] The suggestion here is that an ironic distance can only be achieved after a type of devotion to blood and soil has taken place. In this way, patriotism may not only be "compatible" with irony, it may be its "precondition".[76] After 9/11 this cultural distance may have paved the way for some cringe-worthy and offensive humor, but this humor need not be viewed as un-American or un-patriotic. Indeed it may indicate quite the opposite. Might we not say, therefore, that cringe-worthy or offensive post-9/11 comedy is a patriotic act? Could it be a case of the more offensive the better? If this is the case, then Matt Stone and Trey Parker (the creators of *South Park)* and Seth McFarlane (the creator of *Family Guy* and *American Dad*) are true patriots.

Irony – and its kin metaphor, trope and allegory – is a type of humor that offers an *oppositional double* and, importantly for Kierkegaard, a negation of language.[77] Take, for example, the well-known catch-phrase from *The Crow*[78] – "It can't rain all the time". This phrase is a fine example of irony at work. In one sense, the audience of this ironic phrase might believe that the person who uttered these words has come from a wet climate where a break in the rain would bring relief – chin up! *It can't rain all the time!* Alternatively, for someone from a climate characterized by drought and barren, rainless summers, this ironic phrase takes on a Stoic quality – sure we are in a drought, but *it can't rain all the time!* Irony can coerce its audience to be "both attracted and irritated".[79] Attraction and irritation can be persuasive emotions – when brought together they can be irresistible. Irony, in this way, can compel people to "stay awhile, and ponder, talk, and listen".[80] Milan Kundera believed that irony was irritation, "not because it mocks or attacks but because it denies us our certainties by unmasking the world as an ambiguity".[81]

A special kind of post-9/11 irony permeates the brain-spawn of *Family Guy* and *American Dad* creator Seth McFarlane and *Team American: World Police* and *South Park* creators Matt Stone and Trey Parker. This irony does not mock or attack, but it reveals 9/11 and post-9/11 witnessing as ambiguous, uncertain and emergent. The creators and producers of these programs have been far more active in their participation in post-9/11 tele-visual culture than *The Simpsons'* creators and writers. The programs created by McFarlane, Stone and Parker at times portray stinging criticisms of the post-9/11 world and depict many of 9/11's consequences in hilarious cartoon encounters. Incredibly, McFarlane was almost aboard the plane that was crashed into Tower Two on 9/11. As Griner notes, the nineteen 9/11 hijackers almost played a direct role in how *Family Guy* and *American Dad* would continue to exist after 9/11.[82] As McFarlane describes this day: "Through a combination of me being hung over and being late the next day ... I missed it [American Airlines Flight 11] by 10 minutes. It was very, very fortunate".[83] He added that he would never make jokes about 9/11. McFarlane's ability to make fun of the post-9/11 world given this context would be alarming for some. But perhaps this is the best example yet of the cathartic capacity of laughter. *Family Guy* can be hugely offensive at times, yet in these same moments it can be almost unbearably funny.

Not only did McFarlane go on to make many jokes involving 9/11, he went on to produce a program set definitively in a post-9/11 world. *American Dad* depicts the life and times of CIA agent Stan Smith, "a die-hard Republican obsessed with the threat of terrorism in America".[84] McFarlane describes Stan Smith as the "quintessential post 9/11 paranoid American, who believes everything he hears, and with zero critical thinking, everything is a knee-jerk, angry reaction".[85] Yet, when compared to *Family Guy*, *American Dad* does little to confront 9/11 head-on. Where *Family Guy* made numerous jokes about 9/11 and post-9/11 culture, *American Dad* holds 9/11 as the backdrop for all American culture. Rather than engaging directly with 9/11, the attacks underpin every act, attitude and behavior. The character "Roger" is a particularly allegorical figure in this program. Roger is an alien that was liberated by Stan and his family after he was captured from the crash-landed UFO in Roswell, New Mexico in 1947. By positioning Roger as a focal point in *American Dad*, the writers and producers are making visible a legacy of conspiracy theories, ideas of the military-industrial project, clandestine deals involving the US government and its spooky agencies and a history of covert operations and mistrust of government in this post-9/11 artifact of screen culture. In doing so, *American Dad* sits – strangely – amidst trailblazing science fiction, alien-inspired programs like *X Files*, *The Lone Gunmen* and *Roswell* as well as contemporary cartoons like *Family Guy* and *The Simpsons*.

As a way of cutting through the "mess"[86] left by Seth McFarlane's grappling with the meanings and consequences of the post-9/11 world, I have chosen to focus on some specific episodes of *Family Guy* and *American Dad*. It is the nature of social science mess that some things will be included as knowledge in research and some things will be excluded. There is a distinct possibility that I will exclude something that could be included or include something that could have been excluded, but this is a risk I will have to take. The episodes that I have chosen stood out from others. They are particular signposts in post-9/11 screen cultures. They were episodes that focused specifically on the meanings and consequences of 9/11 and explored with a sense of irony how 9/11 has transformed everyday life.

Seth MacFarlane's Irony – It's Like Two Pies in the Face, and One in a Field in Pennsylvania

Seth MacFarlane's post-9/11 irony is marked by his near miss on 9/11. Due to a late night and an apparent mix up with his travel agent, he avoided dying in the airplane that struck Tower Two. For this reason, one might suspect that he would be unlikely to find the post-9/11 world funny. This is clearly not the case. Seth MacFarlane appeared on *Larry King Live* in April 2010. Larry and Seth discussed what it means to make jokes in the post-9/11 world:

Larry King: Nothing funny that day?

Seth MacFarlane: Nothing funny that day. No, no, no. You know 9/11 was something that – that's an interesting example of something that you don't – you got to pick just the right time to touch it in any kind of humorous way, even if you're making a comment, a satirical comment on the incident and there was a – it was a long time before we felt it was ok and now it's, you know, now it's something that –

Larry: Mel Brookes can do Hitler.

Seth: Yeah, yeah exactly.[87]

Some time was certainly needed. Whilst the initial seasons of *Family Guy* following 9/11 made little reference to the attacks, from season six 9/11 references quickly became a recurring theme – it is a sign that a little distance can create a space for irony and humor. In the season six episode (in the Australian release DVDs) "It Takes a Village Idiot and I Married One", Lois Griffin – Peter Griffin's wife – decides to run for mayor of Quahog vowing not to play the usual political games and engage in mindless rhetoric. She wants to win with a platform of supposedly real issues. With the incumbent Adam West (yes, Adam West of *Batman* fame) leading comfortably in the polls, Lois takes some advice from the family's talking dog, Brian. Brian advises Lois that "undecided voters are the biggest idiots in the world. Try giving short, simple answers"[88] and, wherever possible, appeal to voter's emotions:

Reporter: Sir, your question please?

Man in the audience: Mrs Griffin, what do you plan to do about crime in our city?

Lois: A lot

[crowd cheers]

Lois: Because that's what Jesus wants.

[crowd cheers]

Lois: 9/11 was bad.

[crowd works themselves into a cheering frenzy and some-one mutters "I agree with that"] ...

Man in the audience: Mrs Griffin, what are your plans for cleaning up our environment?

Lois: 9/11

[some of the crowd leaps to its feet and cheers]

Woman in the audience: Mrs Griffin, what about our traffic problem?

Lois: 9 ...

[crowd leans forward in anticipation]

Lois: ... 11

[the entire crowd leaps to its feet in rapture, applauding and cheering].[89]

This theme was similarly depicted in a post-9/11 Doonesbury comic strip published in December 2003. It features a presidential press conference being run by then Whitehouse press secretary, Scott Mc-Clellan. But "Scott never lets a full question get asked".[90]

Reporter: Scott, about the continuing chaos in Iraq

Scott: 9-11

Reporter: Scott, with a half-trillion-dollar deficit, does Bush have

Scott: 9-11

Reporter: Scott, in regard to the ongoing gutting of our envi-ronmental laws

Scott: 9-11

Reporter: Uh ... Scott, is 9-11 the answer to every question now?

Scott: Yes, it's 9-11, 24-7

Reporter: Until when?

Scott: 11-2

Reporter: 10-4.[91]

November 2 was the date of the 2004 US presidential election. This *Doonesbury* comic strip should sound familiar to witnesses of terrorism both inside and outside of the United States. In Australia, we have witnessed a steady stream of major and minor events that have reanimated 9/11 in various guises that cover a broad range of issues ranging from the plight of asylum seekers to the sale of parachutes for office workers that work above the thirteenth floor in tall buildings.[92] The fear that is generated and sustained by 9/11 has forged a powerful political currency. Indeed, fear has long been a powerful political weapon. After 9/11, opportunistic politicians saw 9/11 as a platform on which elections might be won or lost.

In episode one of season eight, "Back to the Woods", Peter Griffin appears on the David Letterman *Tonight Show* impersonating actor James Woods.

> *Letterman*: What are you here to promote James?
>
> *Peter*: Well Dave, I have a hilarious new movie coming out on HBO next month. It's all about 9/11. The movie's called *September 11th, Two Thousand Fun.*
>
> [Letterman's studio audience gasps] …
>
> *Letterman*: James, that sounds unbelievably offensive to Americans.
>
> *Peter*: Well you haven't heard what the movie's about. I play a window washer who has just finished washing the last window on the World Trade Center. And I turn around to get off the scaffold and what do you think I see coming? A plane! And I go "C'MON!". You know, it's real old style comedy, you know, it's like, it's like two pies in the face and one in a field in Pennsylvania.

On the audio commentary for this episode on the 2009 DVD release of season eight of *Family Guy*, one executive producer notes that "A lot of times we make jokes about things that upset us".[93] This is not just about making jokes. This is healing and catharsis through humor. The humor and irony in these scenes is a product of complex social relations and situated audiences. I found these two scenes to be very funny. But the impetus for this humor is tragic and horrific.

All I need to do is glance at the first half of this chapter to feel sad and a little ashamed that I could find these scenes funny.

Among the post-9/11 topics that Seth McFarlane has confronted is the stereotyping of Muslims. In episode seven of season one of *American Dad* titled "Homeland Insecurity", Stan discovers that Iranians have moved to his neighborhood. Stan, as always, overreacts and takes actions towards fighting the "War on Terror" against his neighbors.

> *Francine*: That just leaves the new neighbors
>
> *Stan*: The new neighbors? Memari. Oh God, tell me they're not Italian.
>
> *Francine*: No, I think they're Iranian.
>
> [The Memaris answer the door]
>
> *Stan*: Holy Ayatollah!
>
> *Francine*: Hi. We're your neighbors, Stan and Francine Smith. We came to invite you to our block party.
>
> *Linda*: Oh terrific. Bob and Linda Memari. We'd love to come.
>
> *Stan*: Well maybe some other time. [Francine kicks Stan]. Aggh! So, err, what part of Islam do you hail from.
>
> *Bob*: My parents were from Iran but I was born in Cleveland.
>
> *Stan*: Really? You know we also have a Cleveland here in America and it'd be just super if you didn't blow it up.
>
> *Francine*: So, the block party starts at three and goes till question mark. It's pot luck so bring whatever you want.
>
> *Stan*: But not smallpox. Ha, kidding! Kind of joking, but not really.[94]

This type of racial confusion – where an image of Islam meets the everydayness of human encounters, a place where who is and is not Muslim is deeply problematic[95] – was also satirized in season eight, episode seven of *Family Guy* through the figure of an Indian boy competing in a spelling bee whilst being subjected to discriminatory attitudes from the spelling bee host, recurring character Tom Tucker:

> *Tom*: Our next spelling bee contestant is Omar Muhad-jaree-fa-something September 11th-y
>
> ...
>
> *Tom*: We're now down to our final two competitors. Peter Griffin and Omar North Tower.
>
> ...
>
> *Tom*: [following Omar's misspelling of coagulate] Ooo, I'm sorry Omar. I bet you could spell box-cutters.
> *Omar*: I'm nine-years-old and I'm Indian!

According to Melnick, irrational discrimination and racisms like this have been common in the post-9/11 world. This discrimination might sometimes be directed at Muslims or Arabs. At other times it might be directed at anyone with brown skin, with a particular accent, or anyone dressed a certain way. People that are suspected of being Muslim. There is, perhaps, little consensus on who we are – who is included in and excluded from the category of "we". Surely an Indian boy at a spelling bee is a *we* in reality (on *our* side), but in images he is brown and therefore a potential figure of a terrorist. As legendary African-American rapper KRS-One argued, 9/11 was not a terrorist attack against freedom or democracy, it was an attack on "them down the block".[96] It was an attack on white, wealthy corporate America – Ward Churchill's "little Eichmans".[97] As another Native American author noted: "I am a Native American and therefore have ten thousand more reasons to terrorize the U.S. than any of those Taliban jerk-offs".[98] KRS-One too has a different testimonial of what the destruction of the Twin Towers meant:

> [W]hen we were down at the trade center we were getting hit over the head by cops, told that we can't come in this building ... because of the way we dressed and talked, and so on, we were racially profiled. So, when the planes hit the building we were like mmmm justice.[99]

Once again the complexities and multiplicities of a post-9/11 "we" are revealed. KRS-One did not consider himself victimized by 9/11. He did not consider himself a target. Should we therefore confuse him for a terrorist like some right-wing commentators were want to do after his comments became known?[100]

Seth McFarlane was amongst good comedy-company in picking up on this post-9/11 multiplicity of we. Themes of post-9/11 racism and discrimination in *Family Guy* and *American Dad* were rivaled in hilarity and scathing criticism by some American spy-puppets that police the world.

Matt Stone and Trey Parker's Irony: America! Fuck Yeah!

Matt Stone and Trey Parker are responsible for some of the most scathing political commentary of recent times. From foul-mouthed eight-year-olds in South Park, Colorado to American puppets that police the world, their insights into post-9/11 politics, society and culture can both offend and enlighten. For many of my terrorism studies colleagues, *Team America: World Police* is essential viewing.[101] According to Gow, this film offers "the best vehicle for interpreting and understanding the dominant global security issues of today".[102] *Team America* is set in a post-9/11 world. Its puppet characters are the products of a perpetual terror war and they will not be swayed from their goals to make the world safe from terrorism. But, in the "War on Terror" that Stone and Parker seek to parody, no one ever said the world would be safe from the USA.

Gow believes that the writers' aimed to "balance a presentation of US clumsiness, cultural insensitivity and destructiveness with an interpretation of America's sense of responsibility and good intentions in approaching the world".[103] These heavy-handed good intentions result in the *Team America* spies saving Paris from would-be terrorists at the expense of some of Paris' most iconic landmarks. The message from Parker and Stone is clear – American interventions have the potential to cause more damage than they prevent. But sometimes heavy-handed interventions may be a necessary evil, as the film's crescendo demonstrates. We come to learn that there are three types of people in this world – *dicks, pussies and assholes*. The American attitude towards the world makes them "dicks"; "*We're* reckless, arrogant, stupid dicks".[104] Anti-war activists – epitomized in the film through the *Film Actors Guild*, or *FAG* – are "pussies". International terrorists and leaders of terrorist states are "assholes".

> Pussies don't like dicks because pussies get fucked by dicks. But dicks also fuck assholes. Assholes who just want to shit on everything. Pussies may think they can deal with assholes their way. But the only thing that can fuck an ass-hole is a dick, with some balls. The problem with dicks is that sometimes they fuck too much. Or fuck when it isn't appropriate. And it takes a pussy to show them that. But sometimes pussies get so full of shit that they become ass-holes themselves. Because pussies are only an inch and a half away from assholes. I don't know much in this crazy, crazy world. But I do know that if you don't let us fuck this asshole we are going to have our dicks and our pussies all covered in shit.[105]

It is rare that the problem of responding to terrorism has been stated so paradoxically eloquently and crudely. The lesson is that sometimes people with power should be permitted to crush a de-termined and brutal enemy, but this power must be tempered and blunted. This opens up a variety of possible points of unification in a world that is sometimes divided by the "War on Terror". Could it be that we need *Fox News* like we need the *New York Times*? Do we need ferocious counterterrorism laws to sit alongside political radi-cals and activists? Do we need the binary oppositions of left and right to stand as political departure points for channels of political discourse, such as the ones that are the subject of this chapter? To answer these questions fully I would need many more pages and, perhaps, to be writing a different book. But perhaps it is enough to say that the "War on Terror" is fought on many diverse fronts of which screen cultures are among the most important.

By representing the US's "clumsiness" and "good intentions" *Team America* is positioned in response to the oft asked post-9/11 question, *why do people hate America*? Among the best attempts to answer this question, an attempt that does not resort to claims of simple anti-Americanism and foreign irrationality, is provided in the popular book by Ziauddin Sardar and Merryl Wyn Davies unsurprisingly titled *Why Do People Hate America?*[106] Whilst I am skeptical that America is as widely hated as the authors assume, this book positions tele-visual culture as one of the prime culprits for ire and hate directed towards America. In particular, Sardar and Davies turn their critical attention to the television programs *Alias* and *24*. The authors argue that these programs tell their audiences a great deal about "America and how America sees the world".[107] *Alias'* heroin, the grad-student/superspy Sydney Bristow, is said to embody two personalities, just like the nation she hopes to serve.

> As her *normal* self, she is the personification of innocence and virtue, constantly anxious and insecure, trying hard to improve her college grades, comforting her lovelorn room-mate, lamenting the loss of her fiancé, angry about her alienated father, thinking about her mother, and fending off advances from her goofy reporter friend. There is much introspection, drinking and curling up on overstuffed so-fas, and sensitive and humane exchanges, in her *normal* life. But once she is on a mission, Sydney turns into a fighting machine ... She is totally cool and totally determined, even when villainous interrogators are yanking out one of her molars with pliers.[108]

Whilst I appreciate the authors' hope for an America that would prefer to be "curling up" on the sofa than illegally torturing poten-tial terrorists, I object to the suggestion that the innocent and virtu-ous version of Sydney represents the "normal" version of America. As I have shown in the previous chapter, outbursts of subjective forms of violence are supported by systematic, objective violence. In Jason Bourne's words, *look at what they make you give?* The Ameri-can military had intervened in many theaters of war and conflict well before 9/11 occurred. When, if ever, could we have said that America was the "personification of innocence and virtue". This should not be mistaken for anti-Americanism. This is not a dilem-ma unique to America. The people of most, if not all, nations grap-ple with the meanings and consequences of a violent history. Plus, there is little agreement on what is virtuous and innocent when it comes to thinking about terrorism and global violence. Indeed, this lack of agreement is a cornerstone of terrorism studies scholarship where one person's terrorist is another's freedom fighter.

Yet, framing Sydney as a metaphor for America in this way creates an imagery of an America that would just as sooner steer clear of international affairs, but because of a few low-lifes, dictators and terrorists they are forced to be involved, despite their otherwise better judgment. This is fairly problematic when one considers that even *Fox News'* most caustic right wing commentator, Glenn Beck, believes that the US is far from an innocent observer of world events – indeed, he wishes the US was far less willing to get involved in relationships with dictators and terrorists.[109] Žižek notes how the creators of some of the most popular blockbuster movies including *Batman* and *Spiderman* have gone to great lengths to detail the "uncertainties, weaknesses, doubts, fears and anxieties" of the *superhero* to make them a greater superhero than they first appeared. Sardar and Davies' conceptualization of America alongside Sydney Bristow positions the nation as the superhero, or, perhaps, the world's police. But the irony of such depictions makes the process of creating a superhero farcical:

> In real life, this humanization process undoubtedly reached its apogee in a recent North Korean press release which reported that, at the opening game on the country's first golf course, the beloved president Kim Jong-Il excelled, finishing the entire game of 18 holes in 19 strikes. One can well imagine the reasoning of the propaganda bureaucrat: nobody was going to believe that Kim had managed a hole-in-one every time, so, to make things realistic, let us concede that, just once, he needed two strikes to succeed.[110]

If pop-cultural superheroes have taught us anything we know that with every humanized figure, someone else must be demonized. If the US is the personification of innocence and virtue, then someone else must be the personification of evil and guilt. Stone and Parker regularly take a stab at the idiocy of demonizing a designated Other which, in a post-9/11 world, is invariably in the image of a Muslim. In *Alias*, the enemy takes on many forms, or perhaps *shades*; "Arabs, Chinese, Russians, Cubans", always linked through sinister covert networks.[111] This racist bias that frames the usual suspects as villains, evil-doers and terrorists was cleverly satirized in *Team America* through stereotypical depictions of Muslim terrorists complete with facial scars, Western perceptions of traditional Islamic dress, and a spoof of how Arabic sounds to Western ears where all conversations between Muslim characters involved entirely made-up derivations or conjugations of "Mohammed", "Jihad" and "dhurka".[112]

Sardar and Davies conclude that some American television treats the rest of the world as "essentially America's veranda".[113] Sydney can routinely be seen jettisoning off to all parts only to return to Los Angeles in impossible time. And no matter where Sydney finds herself, "everywhere looks just like Los Angeles, where the show is filmed".[114] Sydney moves through "non-America" like it was America's "backyard".[115] Similarly, viewers of *Team America* were not only informed of the country in which each particular scene was set via a caption, but were also given the number of miles that country was from America – "*Cairo, Egypt – 3000 miles East of America*".[116]

Conclusion: Necessary Laughter

In this conclusion I want to bring the disparate narratives in the first and second halves of this chapter in line with the progressing account of what it means to be a witness of terrorism. I also want to show how comedy and trauma can be more closely linked than they appear at first glance. They are kin, they are companions. One cannot exist without the other, even if they rarely co-exist in the exact same moment. In this chapter I have explored some of the ways that 9/11 and the post-9/11 world have been framed in popular televisual screen culture. I opted to separate this chapter into two distinct yet related narratives – trauma and comedy. The moments of trauma emerged shortly after 9/11. In this time and space people needed to grieve and come to terms with the horror they had witnessed. This was, in many respects, no time for humor. But time heals and it was not long before laughter, and even irony, were possible again. They had not died in the attacks as some had claimed. *The laughter was necessary.* The laughter was cathartic and it showed that healing was possible in the most traumatic circumstances. If this laughter had not occurred, if a post-9/11 silence reigned with people too afraid to speak, smile or laugh, then the terrorists would surely have won.

We should never be silent – silence may lead us down a path where the "War on Terror" could never be won. Yet, as Justin Lewis, Richard Maxwell and Toby Miller point out silence in response to 9/11 was just what some people preferred.[117] In the aftermath of 9/11, White House spokesman Ari Fleischer informed American audiences that they should "watch what they say".[118]

> One of the first casualties in the television war on terrorism was free inquiry on the news and public affairs programs on the major U.S. networks ... Television news and public affairs programming, even the quasi-comedic formats, are the primary means for U.S residents to know the world.[119]

In much the same way that a free press is a cornerstone of democratic life and practice, a certain irony, something akin to a roast, can be a true patriotic act. It would be far less patriotic to suggest that everyone should be silent. Where this silence comes from should perhaps be our most pressing dilemma. As Miller notes, quoting a post 2000 presidential election, on-air conversation between George W. Bush's chief of staff and Judy Woodruff of CNN – "we look forward to working with you".[120] It is not my place to decide whether the chicken or egg comes first.

In Dr Anthony Cordeman's, the Arleigh A. Burke Chair in Strategy at the *Center for Strategic and International Studies* (CSIS), address to the *Global Terrorism Research Centre* (GTReC) in Melbourne in October 2009 he attempted to identify what he described as the "lessons of the Afghan War".[121] It was a fascinating and seemingly honest lecture and discussion – something that I had previously not associated with spokespeople representing American war interests and values. He was critical, reflexive and deeply concerned with finding a way forward in the conflicts in which the US finds itself involved. It prompted me to ask Dr Cordesman a question: did the election of Barack Obama make critical and self-reflexive accounts more likely, or perhaps more possible? He shrugged and said he witnessed no operational change in his spheres of interest. A representative of the US consulate in Melbourne interjected and responded more directly – *feelings towards the US changed overnight.*

Following Obama's election, John Stewart wondered how he would continue to make jokes since he had relied so heavily on making fun of George W. Bush. David Letterman also struggled for appropriate humor in the aftermath of Bush (but through his Cool/Not Cool segment, Bush-as-comedy lived on).[122] The end of Bush's presidency was clearly an opportunity for new beginnings – new comedy, new trauma and a hope that people will once again feel sympathy for America. I am interested in the shapes that patriotic irony will take during the Obama era.

Where does this leave our sociology of "we" and, by extension, where is our witness of 9/11? The problem of witnessing may have reached its epoch with the response to the tragic shootings on 5 November 2009 at Fort Hood military base in Texas. In a moment of national mourning, a time of great sympathy for the US, witnesses were told a tired old story – before opening fire, the Muslim US psychiatrist Nidal Malik Hasan screamed "Allahu Ahkbar!", or God is Great.[123] Let us assume that in the frenzy of an army psychiatrist leaping onto a table and opening fire that "eyewitnesses" were able to clearly discern what he was saying in a foreign language and were therefore certain that he was an Islamic extremist. Let us also assume that despite Army officials being unable to confirm that he had uttered any words before he opened fire and despite a wounded survivor telling his wife that he "didn't say a word", we will soon learn that he was a sinister, covert al-Qaeda operative, waiting as a sleeper for the right moment to attack.[124] Let us also ignore the fact that this may be an entirely unfounded claim since, as audiences of terror, we have yet to see anything other than a journalistic report. Let us assume that Nidal Malik Hasan is a terrorist of the highest order. Even if we believe all of these things, to sustain this belief we must also ignore the fact that this is not the first time that a US soldier has become violent and turned the gun against colleagues, comrades and civilians to devastating effect. We would also have to ignore the fact that this attack at least partly simulates that famous scene from Stanley Kubrick's *Full Metal Jacket*.[125] We must also pretend, on some level, that if this was a white American who had committed this atrocity we should be, somehow, surprised. We are told to pretend that a Muslim carrying out such an attack is routine.

A forgetful culture is not a patriotic culture. A forgetful culture will not be endeared to the world, but such a culture may be fertile for resentment, anger and blowback. Bill O'Reilly engages in such forgetfulness when he accuses guests of engaging in extreme left-wing ideologies when they point out that the US once supported the Mujahideen in Afghanistan in the 1980s. Dan Rather engages in this forgetfulness when he suggests that Americans could not possibly understand how a group of people could attack another. Sam Seeborn is forgetful when he suggests that terrorism always fails. John Stewart, Seth McFarlane, Matt Stone and Trey Parker, and the creators of *The Simpsons* are discernibly less forgetful.

James Der Derian has interpreted this forgetfulness as a *"new imbalance of terror"*.[126] This imbalance emerges from systemic and institutionalized "mimetic fear and hatred" combined with an "asymmetrical willingness and capacity to destroy the other without the formalities of war".[127] Der Derian has something more literal in mind I think with this second phrase, but his words are also relevant as a metaphor for my tasks in this book. The ability to destroy the Other without the formality of war – to inflict a symbolic death – is a core contingency of much of the screen cultures featured in this chapter and throughout this book. But this symbolic death did not extend – thankfully – to comedy, irony, and certainly not to trauma.[128] Der Derian seems to have it right when he concludes that "the weapon of mass whimsy might still be the best way to counter the mimetic war of images".[129]

7.

Terrorsex
Witnesses, Spectacular Terrorism and Pornography

I'm used to it! Y'know, like cafeteria food, or the constant threat of terrorism.[1]

An image, I believe, affects us directly, below the level of representation: at the level of intuition, of perception. At that level, the image is always an absolute surprise. At least it should be.[2]

You're only as good as your fans.[3]

We are all witnesses.[4]

It has often been quipped that "9/11" changed the world forever. The unspoken meaning of this phrase lies in the fact that 9/11 was *witnessed* as an image by millions of people throughout the world. Some were witnesses in real-time, some were witnesses from a distance, and some were witnesses as part of a television audience. Many more people were witnesses of the devastating and remarkable consequences of 9/11 – two bloody international wars, the curving of freedoms and liberties in democratic countries, abuse and discrimination directed at people perceived to be Muslim, and widespread fear and anxiety. Being a witness of 9/11 and its consequences myself – in real-time in my bedroom in Geelong, Australia on the evening of 9/11, just after 10pm Australian Eastern Standard

Time with first reports rolling in as I watched *West Wing* — provoked me to ask some fundamental questions about the meanings of terrorism, the meanings of witnessing, the meanings of television images, the meanings of spectacular violence, and – eventually – how I came to understand what I saw as the unexpected yet powerful links between terrorism and pornography.[5]

On 9/11 witnesses were voyeurs. When witnesses of terrorism are viewed in such a way terrorism becomes a shocking and horrific occurrence that is laced with phantasmic enjoyment, or *jouissance*, and, oddly, intense pleasure and gratification. Yet, it is also a site for intense anxiety and the terror and disgust that is always associated with a full and traumatic realization of a fantasy. Pornography can achieve this, but 9/11 achieves this in a particular way. As Kay argues of pornography:

> Pornography is split between maintaining narrative (usually comic or absurd) and graphically portraying sexual activity, always losing sight of one or the other; in its desperate attempt to "show it all", pornography reveals its incapacity to do so… pornography commands the gaze; the presence of the camera, far from disturbing our enjoyment, enables it, since it includes us within the shameless picture.[6]

In this chapter I will frame the voyeur as a producer as well as a consumer of the spectacle of terrorism. Žižek argues that the voyeur is always stained on the image or scene that they witness.[7] As witnesses of 9/11 were we far from passive – we were active, we engaged, we inscribed meaning and consequence, we were voyeurs in the 9/11 (and post-9/11) house of horrors.

Of course these issues are not novel and in struggling to understand these forces (witnessing, spectacular terrorism, global audiences of violent images in the theater of terrorism, terrorism's pornographic qualities) I make reference to a particular tradition of critical thought that has explored the meanings and consequences of terrorism alongside the meanings and consequences of pornography. In the sections that follow I provide an overview of this critical thought as well as the work of some other critical theorists with something important to say about terrorism to position the role of the witness in understanding the meanings and consequences of what I call *terrorsex* – spectacular terrorism as pornography. Drawing on this literature and representations of terrorsex in two screen cultural mediums, I will explore the uncanny links that fuse terrorism with pornography, a fusion that I argue to be the essence of *terrorsex*.[8] Terrorsex represents a crucial moment where terrorism can be understood as a product of *witnesses, spectacles, violence, consumable images, pop-culture, the globalized news media, pornography and voyeurism*. Lurking just beneath these forces are fragile, fearful, precarious and vulnerable human beings living in a world that can be indefinitely described as post-9/11.

The Pornography of Terrorism

There is a surprisingly abundant literature that has explored the links between terrorism and pornography. Much of this literature is provided by critical theorists engaging in what might be described as *critical sociologies of terrorism*, but they are not alone in their accounts of terrorsex. Canonical terrorism studies academics have found use for comparisons between terrorism and pornography. When these links are explored these theorists are not necessarily referring to graphic depictions of sex. Rather, they are suggesting that terrorism and pornography are powerfully, and perhaps unexpectedly, linked. Harvard University terrorism studies academic Louise Richardson argues that "Like pornography, we know terrorism when we see it".[9] Well-known terrorism theorist Walter Laqueur has argued that linking terrorism with pornography may be a way to overcome disputes over the meanings and definitions of terrorism. He argued that "the absence of an exact definition does not mean that we do not know in a general way what terrorism is; it has been said that it resembles pornography, difficult to describe and define, but easy to recognize when one sees it".[10] Reuter offered support to this idea when he quipped that "Most people end up taking a similar approach to terrorism as they do to pornography: I cannot define it, but I know it when I see it".[11] But these links between pornography and terrorism perhaps pose more questions than they answer: do we really know terrorism when we see it? Do we know pornography when we see it?

To understand these questions it is important to understand that the relationship between terrorism and pornography is far more complex than "seeing is believing". It is a relationship that is a product of intersecting forces that include the spectacular violence of terrorism; television and a global media audience; cycles of war, poverty and oppression in third world countries; and the idiosyncratic cultural and social conditions of the witnesses who experience the emotion called *terror*. People who feel terror do not necessarily need to be living and working in close proximity to terrorist violence. Terrorism transcends the time and space in which it first occurs by being captured as tele-visual images that can be replayed over and over again. The visual power of spectacular terrorism sets in motion powerful forces that have played significant roles in war, politics, and society. Indeed this was undoubtedly the 9/11 terrorists' goal – they wanted people watching their horrific violence, not just corpses.

When viewed in this context pornography should be understood as symbolizing a type of transparency and an over-exposure between the "viewer and viewed"[12], a deletion of the symbolic distance between the voyeur and the image, and the embodiment of a really existing *simulation* of violence. In its most common usage pornography is graphic images and tele-visual depictions of sexual acts that provide voyeurs – the witnesses – stimulation and gratification. Some theorists have suggested that terrorism functions at a comparable level working best when it is captured by cameras that transmit graphic images to audiences of witnesses – the voyeurs – who are also the terrorists' living targets.[13] Terrorism viewed in this way is theater for the living – those who die in terror attacks are instruments to that end.

Merrin[14] describes this transparency and over-exposure as "the "pornography" of the real". He argues that pornography's "motivating phantasy is reality".[15] It makes the fractured, disorienting and complex images of *reality* hypervisible, hyperknowable and "dominated"[16] by a "vertiginous phantasy of exactitude". Baudrillard described this as an "*orgy of realism, an orgy of production*".[17] Indeed, Merrin's exploration of the "pornography of the real" owes much to Baudrillard's seminal work on the notion of "hyperreality". For Baudrillard hyperreality is a "real without origin or reality".[18] The term is most often deployed by Baudrillard's followers to explain media – particularly news media – imagery. Baudrillard himself deployed hyperreality in such a way in his controversial book *The Gulf War Did Not Take Place*.[19] As the title suggests, he argued that the first Gulf War never occurred despite embedded journalists beaming images of war directly into the world's televisions. In a sense, he really did mean that the war never occurred. In another sense, Baudrillard was offering a critique of the news media and what it means to witness something that is real. For Baudrillard media images should not be judged on whether they are true or false, real or unreal. They are better than reality, they improve reality and capture it in a seemingly objective medium – in short, media images are *hyperreal*. Whilst we may rightly accept that the first Gulf War did occur – since we are forced to have an unwavering faith in images – Baudrillard forced us to confront the fact that the way we came to learn about the Gulf War was, mostly, dependant on media imagery.[20] Hyperreality forces us to question how we know – was the reporting of the Gulf War real, or was it a *simulation*? Baudrillard suggested with the concept of hyperreality that it is both and that the distinction between reality and simulations was problematic at best, inconsequential at worst.

Perhaps predictably, Baudrillard deployed the notion of hyperreality to explore the meanings of 9/11 and he again decided that they never occurred.[21] This was also where the connections he found between 9/11 and pornography began to emerge. These connections are grounded in the powerful but problematic links between images and their witnessing. Baudrillard argued that 9/11 was the ultimate event, the "mother" of all events, albeit of events that never really took place. Or, stated differently, events that take place as an image-event, a simulated act of violence on television, a hyperreal event.[22] 9/11 was consumed by images, and the images were in turn consumed by media audiences – their "universal attraction" to terrorism is, according to Baudrillard, "on a par with pornography".[23] Terrorism and pornography attract attention by bringing about excesses – excesses of reality, excesses of obscenity, excesses of response, excesses of exposure.[24]

These excesses can have significant consequences. I want to summarize the nature of these consequences through a metaphor provided by Žižek writing about the meanings and consequences of 9/11:

> Is not the ultimate figure of the passion for the Real the option we get on hardcore websites to observe the inside of a vagina from the vantage point of a tiny camera at the top of a penetrating dildo? At this extreme point, a shift occurs: when we get too close to the desired object, erotic fascination turns into disgust at the Real of the bare flesh.[25]

At what point does graphic pornography become little more than a film to educate medical students? At what point does 9/11 become little more than a parody of obscene violence? Žižek's conceptualization forces us to confront the possibility that we saw too much of 9/11, far more than we wanted to. This is the context for Žižek's and Baudrillard's contention that witnesses had fanticized about 9/11 long before it occurred. For Žižek and Baudrillard this was evidenced by the constant stream of disaster films produced in Hollywood depicting end-of-the-world scenarios before 9/11. Indeed, they argue that we had been desensitized. When 9/11 occurred, witnesses could not help but lust after the image-violence that was depicted in the disaster films that were box office mega-hits in so many parts of the world. Or, as Baudrillard argued, "they *did* it, but we *wished for* it".[26]

Ignatieff adds that terror pornography had been a key goal for terrorists that "have been quick to understand that the camera has the power to frame a single atrocity and turn it into an image that sends shivers down the spine of an entire planet".[27]

> This is terrorism as pornography, and it acts like pornography: at first making audiences feel curious and aroused, despite themselves, then ashamed, possibly degraded and finally, perhaps, just indifferent. The audience for this vileness is global. A Dutchman who runs a violent and sexually explicit Web site that posts beheadings notes, in his inimitable words, that "during times of tragic events like beheadings," his site, which usually gets 200,000 visitors a day, gets up to 750,000 hits.[28]

This type of viewing is something akin to rubber necking at a car accident – no one should want to see it, but we are nonetheless compelled to watch. This compulsion has reached dramatic proportions on Australian television. In an article in Melbourne's *The Age* newspaper, Ziffer considers the popularity of one of Australia's top-rating television shows, *Border Security: Australia's Front Line*.[29] This is television for the post-9/11 consumer "where anonymous customs officials are top-rating television stars as Australia tunes in to terror television".[30] I was interviewed for Ziffer's article and I made the point that *Border Security* represents Australia's "national security obsession". Watching this show "fulfils a real fascination, but it also has a sickly attraction, like pornography".[31] When considered in this way, the key to understanding the meanings and nature of pornography will perhaps have little to do with sex.

This idea is well supported in the critical theory/pornography literature. Toffoletti, for example, argues (following Dworkin and MacKinnon) that pornography is "fundamentally concerned" with "a practice of representation".[32] Pornography is a crisis of representation where the "distance implied by the gaze gives way to an instantaneous, exacerbated representation".[33] This view was shared by Baudrillard:

> The only phantasy in pornography, if there is one, is thus not a phantasy of sex, but of the real, and its absorption into something other than the real, the hyperreal. Pornographic voyeurism is not a sexual voyeurism, but a voyeurism of representation and its perdition, a dizziness born of the loss of the scene and the irruption of the obscene.[34]

I use this non-sexual pornography as conceptualized by Baudrillard as a point of departure for my sometimes non-sexual pornography of terrorism. Terror porn is a crisis of representation, not of sex. As I will demonstrate later in this chapter, however, terror and sex may not be so distantly related and there may be little need to distinguish between terrorism and pornography.

Present in pornography in all its forms is *obscenity*. Pornography stands apart from more benign imagery because it is obscene.

> Obscenity is not confined to sexuality, because today there is a pornography of information and communication, a pornography of circuits and networks, of functions and objects in their legibility, availability, regulation, forced signification, capacity to perform, connection, polyvalence, and their free expression. It is no longer the obscenity of the hidden, the repressed, the obscure, but that of the visible, all-too-visible, the more visible than visible; it is the obscenity of that which no longer contains a secret and is entirely soluble in information and communication.[35]

But the odd thing about pornography despite its crisis of overrep-resentation, or over-exposure, is that it is not the real thing, and it will never be as good as the *real thing*. As such pornographic im-agery sits amongst other consumable commodities identified by Žižek where the "product is deprived of its substance" but retains a "hard resistant kernel of the real".[36] Pornography is another in a series of commodities that embody an absence: things that are "deprived of their malignant properties" (like milk and cream without fat).[37] Pornography, to the voyeur, is not real sex. It is an image-based, simulated sex – real enough, perhaps. The witnesses of terrorism in Melbourne on 9/11, where I conducted the research I report on in chapter two, never viewed terrorism as the real thing. It was violence as an image. It was violence without violence. It was the pornography of terrorism – *terrorsex*. Only a small percentage of 9/11's witnesses watched the violence as a "real" event. The vast majority witnessed the event as hyperreality on television.

Case Studies in Terrorsex

Baudrillard once wrote that "Sex is everywhere".[38] Since 9/11, the same can be said of terrorism. The 9/11 terrorist attacks have been replayed again and again on television and the internet (where the destruction of the Twin Towers is a "Google" away) and reanimated to contextualize the latest terror scare. Whether in popular culture, on television, in newspapers, on the Internet or in the minds of a distant audience of witnesses, images of terrorism at critical moments in time and space appear and reappear in routine and banal ways. In particular, cityscapes are a place where terrorism as spectacle – the attraction to which is akin to pornography – becomes attractive to the voyeur of images of terrorism. The fusion of terror and sex through encounters of embodied humiliation, damage and destruction – such as that which occurred on 9/11 and in many theaters since 9/11 – forges in witnesses a sickly desire to watch. Humiliation, damage, death and devastation are routine features of Hollywood disaster movies, and they were routine features on 9/11, and were again on several occasions following 9/11 such as in a *Vogue: Italia* fashion shoot, in Abu Ghraib prison in Iraq, and in a popular television show called *Dollhouse*. But where Hollywood disaster fiction is mere violent pornography, 9/11 and its aftermath is on a par with snuff pornography – a gritty and horrific real pornography.

Strike a National Security Pose

Terrorism produces tantalizing images that possess the ability to shock and cause horror. People seemingly cannot help but watch. This was the context for Richardson when she writes that terrorism is like pornography in that we know it when we see it.[39] This was what was at stake in the case of the fusion of terror and sex in a photo spread published in *Vogue: Italia* in 2006. These photographs depict banal, routine and mundane sexual situations at critical moments of anti-terrorism and security – a skinny, blonde model splayed against a car being searched in a sexually aggressive manner by a counterterrorism police officer in riot gear, another forced into an excruciating pose with pressure point techniques administered by air marshals and another of a routine strip search at an airport check point. The embodied humiliation is completed with airport security guards acting as voyeurs. Here, images structure a post-9/11 terror porn fantasy. But such images need to be more than just spectacular, they also need to be banal and everyday to truly capture the attentions of witnesses in everyday ways. Witnesses are consumed by banal routines and the spectacular functions as a temporary intervention. The everyday, however, stays with us and cannot be left behind.

According to Baudrillard, what people desire most when watching pornography and terrorism is the "spectacle of banality".[40]

The spectacle of banality is today's true pornography and obscenity. It is the obscene spectacle of nullity, insignificance, and platitude. This stands as the complete opposite of the theatre of cruelty. But perhaps there is still a form of cruelty, at least a virtual one, attached to such a banality. At a time when television and the media in general are less and less capable of accounting for the world's (unbearable) events, they rediscover daily life.[41]

Perhaps this is the reason that counterterrorism and security is the theme of one of Australia's highest rating television programs *Border Patrol*. Or why the drama series 24 rates highly all over the world, and why people flocked to blockbuster disaster movies based on the 9/11 terrorist attacks complete with real flight crew as actors.[42] They all represent the ushering of terrorism into the everyday as a way of routinizing these otherwise unbearable world events. Perhaps it is also why the editors at *Vogue: Italia* believed that a national security theme fused with banal pornography was a good way to promote their fashion lines. In the post-9/11 world,[43] 9/11 is reanimated, reconstituted, and re-depicted in images that simulate violence and offer it for consumption: this, I argue, is the *commodification of terrorsex*.

The commodity of terrorsex can be illustrated by juxtaposing contrasting images. The first image is an advertisement from *Dolce & Gabbana*, commonly referred to as the "gang rape" advertisement, where five skinny yet muscular men and a woman are featured in a pre-gang rape scenario.[44] The woman is held down by the wrists by one of the attackers while she raises her hips in the air as a form of timid resistance. Four other men stand watching in everyday poses. The exposed part of their bodies glisten and the whole scene appears to be atop a tall building somewhere in a city. The advertisement was pulled after protestations from women's rights groups but this did not prevent one commentator from wondering "Is the image glorifying gang rape or tapping into a sexual fantasy?"[45] Possibly even an "erotic dream" or a "sexual game".[46] The second image is the most mundane and routine of scenarios. Five young men and women sit chatting on a sunny morning next to a body of water.[47] They appear relaxed, comfortable and jovial. In the background, smoke billows from the island of Manhattan as the Twin Towers burn. I suggest that these photographs can be viewed as a reminder that spectacular events such as pack rape and terrorism can be depicted as everyday parts of life in the city, and their occurrence as banal, everyday and routine.

Images of terrorism, counterterrorism and post-9/11 security have also become part of the everyday so perhaps these images are not as abhorrent and shocking as they first appear. But then again, this is also their diabolical nature. Perhaps we *should* find images such as these disturbing and something that is not routine. In a particularly routine and spectacular attempt to capture post-9/11 pornography, the editors of *Vogue: Italia* repackaged national security through gendered and embodied images in the fetishistic pursuit of terrorsex. These images combine the routinized surveillance of traveling through airports with the hetero-erotic spy fantasies depicted in Hollywood blockbusters. Spy-chic has a history littered with promiscuous superbabes encoded through bisexual suggestion and paradoxical power and subservience. *Charlie's Angels*,[48] played by Cameron Diaz, Lucy Liu and Drew Barrymore, are powerful, dangerous and threatening women, yet they are the security hand-maidens of Bosley: they can be viewed in this way as the ultimate weapon of a patriarch. *La Femme Nikita*[49] was the street kid encoded as risky and untamed until exchanging imprisonment for national servitude as an assassin: her transformation invoked images of man as the savior of the female body in much the same way that it was depicted in *Pretty Woman*.[50] Sexualized images of security are perhaps best captured by the Bond women: always stunning, sexually promiscuous (a concept satirized in *Austin Powers: The Spy Who Shagged Me*[51] through Felicity Shagwell), and often treacherous. The Bond women have often turned on 007 at the earliest convenience as double agents and enemies of the state. This theme was powerfully captured in *Casino Royale* through the supposedly empowered feminist, Vesper Lynd.[52]

The *Vogue: Italia* photographs are "sexual and odd, but also quite mundane, quite familiar".[53] The set of photographs contain pictures of women as both terrorists and counterterrorists: the terrorists are forced into painful and humiliating poses whilst the counterterrorists are splayed in various poses whilst receiving training from square-jawed men who are seemingly not distracted by the exceedingly tall, skinny, and glamorous women clinging to large automatic and semi-automatic weapons and laden down with extravagantly applied mascara and eyeliner. The first photograph features a "rake-skinny, plague-pallored model" removing her skirt revealing tight, black underwear seemingly at the command of the voyeuristic security guards (one woman, one man, another unidentifiable).[54]

The scene creates the impression that, for what could be a number of reasons in this security obsessed world, she has been stopped at a security checkpoint and has been asked to remove her clothes. She does so sternly yet submissively: she makes the necessary sacrifice and we watch. In another, a blonde woman is pressed face-down on a road with two security police: one pointing a gun at her from a few feet away, the other grabbing her hair and applying pressure to the back of her head with one hand and holding her wrists behind her back with the other, his thigh nestled between her parted legs. She is wearing a flimsy and silky dress that resembles a lace negligee, and her latté lies spilt on the road beside her.

Another photograph features a woman in a bright red dress with a police boot on her throat and a police shield slid between here closed but partly exposed thighs. In another, a tall and skinny woman stands with her hands on the roof of a police car while a riot-cop hitches up her dress as part of a body search.

Two images, in particular, immediately grabbed my attention and are powerful representations of terrorsex. The first of these photographs features a woman at an airport security screening machine, her shirt draped over the conveyor-belt as she stands with arms and legs outstretched wearing a bra that covers only part of her breasts and a skirt that ends just before her knees. A female security guard, queered with a tightly worn hair-bun, a button-down shirt and slacks, rests one hand on her stomach as she scans her left breast with a hand-held metal detector. A male security guard carries on his regular duties apparently without noticing the sexualized security occurring only a short distance away. It is for this male security guard so mundane, so banal, and so everyday: a routine scene in the post-9/11 world. The woman is compelled into nudity as national security demands. The love affair between the witness and the image is most diabolical in this sexualized, gendered and embodied form. To the heading "Nothing Sexy About Nude Scans", the Associated Press reports of new technology soon to be commonplace in the world's airports that allows security screeners to see under the clothes of travelers.[55] A spokeswoman for the manufacturers explained that the images produced are "kind of futuristic. There's nothing sexy about it".[56] Not unsexy enough however for *The Age* newspaper to publish a front-on image of the scan, preferring instead to show one of a muscular male from behind. In early 2010, these scanners returned to prominence in the media following the attempted Christmas Day terror attack on a commercial airplane as it approached Detroit.[57] Much to the chagrin of civil liberties and human rights groups, these security measures are expected to become standard throughout many of the world's airports amid assurances that the technology will not be used inappropriately. Again, nudity appears in the same space as counterterrorism in another bizarre twist in the post-9/11 "war" on the emotion called "terror".

The second photograph features a skinny and heavily made-up woman on her knees with her hands behind her head. Some of her belongings lay scattered beside her. Two security guards stand before her and the whole scene appears to be in an airport. One security guard holds a baton in a quasi-threatening manner – perhaps representing the uncertainty and ambiguity of counterterrorism security operations, not prepared to strike, not prepared to put the baton away – whilst another holds an aggressive German Shepherd attack dog baring its teeth, barking and preparing to strike at the hapless woman. The scene immediately resonates (as I believe it is meant to) with the horrific images of abuse carried out by US soldiers in the notorious Abu Ghraib prison in Iraq.[58]

As Johnston opines, perhaps all that was needed to complete the pictures in *Vogue: Italia* were electrical wires and a hood to further emulate the images of torture of detainees by American soldiers at Abu Ghraib.[59] The eroticized and pornographic replication of Abu Ghraib is unmistakable. Susan Sontag insisted that the images of Abu Ghraib were pornographic through the depictions of masturbation, oral sex, nudity, and humiliation.[60] Žižek believes that the Abu Ghraib torture and abuse points to an underlying malaise in

American culture. He argues that the "main feature that strikes the eye" in viewing the Abu Ghraib torture images is the difference between the "standard" way that prisoners were tortured under Saddam Hussein's government and the torture prisoners were subjected to under US military occupation.[61] Under Saddam the focus of torture was physical, under US occupation the focus of torture was "psychological humiliation".[62] This combined with the recording of the torture with a digital camera, its decisively (homo)sexual dimensions, and its theatrical staging make the Abu Ghraib torture all the more visible, graphic and shocking. Much like they did for 9/11, the images and reality of the spectacular violence combined to create something more horrific than the images or reality alone. As such, the Abu Ghraib images sit alongside the *Vogue: Italia* images as an overwhelmingly pure representation of terrorsex.

According to Mirzoeff, what viewers witness in the Abu Ghraib images is "sodomy … visualized as embodied spectacle".[63] This idea is meticulously studied (among other related subjects) by Jasbir Puar.[64] She argues that with Abu Ghraib a line was crossed, a line marked at a point of demarcation when routine torture (a torture that Puar considers an everyday part of US culture) makes way for sex torture; a torture designed to "mimic sexual acts closely associated with deviant *sexuality* or *sexual excess* such as sodomy and oral sex, as well as S/M practices of bondage, leashing, and hooding".[65] The notion of sexual excess captures the pornographic obscenity and intent of the Abu Ghraib amateur film-makers. This was the basis of Baudrillard's description of the images of Abu Ghraib torture as "War Porn".[66] As Baudrillard contextualized this argument:

> September 11th, the exhilarating images of a major event; in the other [Abu Ghraib images], the degrading images of something that is the opposite of an event, a non-event of an obscene banality, the degradation, atrocious but banal, not only of the victims, but of the amateur scriptwriters of this parody of violence.[67]

For Baudrillard, the pornography of war is an "illustration of a power which, reaching its extreme point, no longer knows what to do with itself – a power henceforth without aim, without purpose, without a plausible enemy, and in total impunity".[68] My goal here is not to bombard the US military with criticism and insult – there are many who have done this better than I could. My goal is to bring to the surface the ways that this power has become pornographic and ushered in moments of terrorsex. The Abu Ghraib torture images clearly represent such a moment – it has powerfully captured the pornography of terrorism and the pornography of unmediated power (unmediated, that is, until the image takes off and saturates witnesses throughout the world).

In this way the images of Abu Ghraib are not only pornographic through their depictions of sexual depravity, but also through the over-exposure and the confrontation with an image that shows too much that witnesses must endure. Indeed, some argue that images such as Abu Ghraib are more than merely pornographic. The Abu Ghraib images, perhaps, have more in common with "snuff movies" and "gonzo porn" where the depravity is not simulated as it is in many pornographic films. Via mini-cams, digital photography and camera phones everyone is potentially a director of obscenity. As a consequence of this a new type of porn emerges: "(pornography) is much, much dirtier than it used to be, but Gonzo porno is gonzo: way out there. The new element is violence".[69] "Gonzo" was initially used to refer to the journalism of Hunter S. Thompson who made himself an implicit part of the story he was covering. This usually involved hedonistic behavior particularly involving drug use. More recently it has been used to describe a genre of pornography: the gritty and unpolished look makes amateur porn feel more real to the voyeur.[70] It is not glossed with sophisticated production methods: it is the image laid bare, providing the witness with the phantastic belief that it represents a more grounded image than Hollywood fiction can provide.

Viewed in this context the *Vogue: Italia* images represent something deeply obscene about contemporary visual culture. Digital cameras are everyday tools of life found as both regular cameras and conveniently in mobile phones and digital organizing systems. Internet news outlets gain almost immediate access through community informants and data mining on weblogs and Internet diaries. In no other time have the private lives of people been so consumable, such a commodity, so real. This is what Sontag was describing when she argued that each person is the master of "his or her own reality show".[71] For some American soldiers, this reality show was gonzo pornography. Every aspect of life is recordable and can be disseminated to all parts of the world, and more people tend to watch when this everydayness descends into "crisis and disgrace".[72] The images generated by such a crisis become the tool of marketers, politicians, and academics. The torture at Abu Ghraib is witnessed more because it was a sexual act. These photos of torture were found in a camera that had captured many other images of American soldiers in Iraq, images that included soldiers engaging in sexual acts. War-porn. Terror-porn. As if images of war and terror were not explicit or perverse enough.

The Abu Ghraib images occupy a space between porn and terror. It is a unique blend that was perhaps sure to attract the camera's attention as what Johnson describes as "grainy spectacles of terror".[73] Through Abu Ghraib and *Vogue: Italia* images of 9/11 are reanimated. They are consumable post-9/11 images of terror. The terrorists on 9/11 and their collaborators are as much amateur directors choreographing a feature film to enthral a generation as were the US soldiers at Abu Ghraib. We look, we watch, we see. Then we replay and watch again and again. The splayed legs of the models in *Vogue: Italia* are a metaphor for the disintegrating Twin Towers. They are images of punishment and retribution and of humiliation and terror. The witness is the voyeur in this black museum.[74]

Inside the Dollhouse: Post-9/11 Whores and Secret Agents

> Children are fascinated with dollhouses, perhaps because each represents a miniature fantasy world with so much to think about and do: assign dolls to rooms, arrange furniture, create accessories from found items, discuss relationships between dolls, and act out dramas to satisfy the dolls' (and owners') feelings.[75]

The Joss Whedon created television series *Dollhouse* tells the story of "Caroline/Echo" and her entry into a world of contracted servitude for a shady and mysterious corporation—*Rossum Corporation*[76]—with an agenda for global domination. The story begins when

"Caroline" — an anti-globalization activist — is captured after break-
ing into their hidden underground compound. The first scene in the
first episode of season one shows Caroline being offered a choice
– she can receive her punishment, which the viewer is encouraged
to assume may be death, or she can sign the contract that is placed
in front of her. This contract contains the terms and conditions for
Caroline becoming a "doll" for a period of five years. Under the
terms of the contract her memory will be wiped and returned to
her when her contract ends. She will work with clients who have
purchased her services. These clients will provide the criteria for a
new set of memories, a new personality, that will be temporarily
uploaded into her memory-void. At the end of each mission, her
memory will again be wiped. When her contract is finished, her
debt repaid, she will be free to leave with her original memories
returned to her. Until then she is a blank slate, a *doll*. As a doll she is
to leave "Caroline" behind. She begrudgingly agrees, and is labeled
with the designation "Echo".

Unsurprisingly, the show delves into a variety of ethical issues
– the meanings of humanity and post-humanity; mind-body dual-
isms; spirituality and the soul; and crime and punishment, to name
a small few. The writers of *Dollhouse* are eager to frame the show in
these ethical terms in the first episode. The following dialogue takes
place between the scientist who developed the brain programming
and replacing technology, Topher, and Echo's "handler", Boyd – a
person who cares for Echo before, during and after missions. They
are discussing Echo's recent mission in which she was a weekend
sexual fling for a wealthy client:

> *Topher*: The new moon has made her virgin again … She had
> fun right?
> *Boyd*: She thought so.
> *Topher*: There is nothing good or bad but thinking makes
> it so, man-friend. We gave two people a perfect weekend
> together. We're great humanitarians.
> *Boyd*: Who'd spend their lives in jail if anyone found this
> place [the Dollhouse].[77]

Indeed, the difference between a criminal and a humanitarian– and, as we come to learn, between a whore and a secret agent – is a fine one. The Dollhouse director – Adelle Dewitt – tells Caroline that her desire to help others can be realized in the Dollhouse – sometimes as a whore, sometimes as a secret agent, but always as a humanitarian. Yet Caroline's humanitarian "choice" is a false one: *be a good humanitarian, or die.*

For Joss Whedon (a "godlike" figure amongst tele-visual "geeks"[78]) *Dollhouse* is not about humanitarianism; it is about "fantasies": "When you're dealing with fantasies, particularly sexual ones, you're going off the reservation. You're not going to be doing things that are perfectly correct. It's supposed to be about the sides of us that we don't want people to see".[79] It is these fantasmic coordinates of *Dollhouse* that allows it to sit comfortably in a post-9/11 world as an artifact of terrorsex. *Dollhouse* agents inevitably play one of two roles – they are either *whores or secret agents*. It is yet another post-9/11 commodity of terrorsex.

Patterson frames the character Caroline/Echo as a "sort-of Stepford wife, a not-quite Nikita" or a "Narcissus-type nymph".[80]

> Prostitution is indeed on the bill. Echo functions as a classy motorcycle-racing escort, as an outsdoorsy rock-climbing escort, as a thief pretending to be a trashy thigh-high-boot-wearing escort. But her superiors also, for some reason, seem to program her as an Alpine midwife, and she has great potential as a killing machine.[81]

This is Caroline's/Echo's lot in life as long as she is contracted to the mysterious *Rossum Corporation*. Alarmingly, Echo proves to be unique. Viewers soon learn that when she is wiped at the end of each mission, she retains certain memories that are ultimately re-animated in other missions – often to help her survive. There have been times when Echo has been playing a role as an escort only to find herself in a dangerous predicament. When faced with danger she has been able to call on martial arts and weapons training that she was programmed with during previous missions when she was a secret agent. As a result she becomes an aberration and the ultimate sexual killing machine. Yet she is no-one at the same time. She can be seen asking anyone who will listen, "Do you know which one is real?"

When Echo is not having kinky sex with a client, she is often employed alongside the FBI or the ATF as a specialist agent. In episode five of season one titled "True Believer" Echo is recruited by the FBI to infiltrate a religious cult in order to beam back images of what is happening in their "Waco-style"[82] compound:

> *Senator Boxbaum*: We're talking about people here who have their very wills taken away.
>
> *Adelle Dewitt*: Imagine such a thing.
>
> *Senator*: The irony of bringing this to you, Adelle, is not lost on me. I promise you.
>
> *Adelle*: It's not the irony that concerns me. You're asking me to place an Active with a federal agent.
>
> *Senator*: Indirectly, yes.
>
> *Adelle*: I don't wish to be vulgar, but one of the many benefits of having you as a client is that you help us avoid entanglements with federal agencies.
>
> *Senator* (chuckling): It's the ATF. You been running guns? Besides, your Actives won't be working with the government. One of your security guys would liaise. Your Active would be perfectly safe.
>
> *Adelle*: In a fanatical religious cult?
>
> *Senator*: Adelle ... This is an election year.
>
> *Adelle*: Ah.
>
> *Senator*: I got the family value voters on the right, the women's issues constituency on the left all coming after me if anything untoward is going on behind those compound walls. The ATF is convinced there is. Now, we have a very narrow window on this warrant. If the government sends in some wet-behind-the-ears Quantico undercover graduate, these people are gonna know about it. I need the real thing. I need a *true believer*.[83]

Senator Boxbaum's desire for the "real thing" produces an Echo programmed as a blind traveler who is devoted to the teachings of this religious cult whose members are suspected of criminal activities. She is embedded into the service of the federal government not as a spy; she is something quite different, something much more authentic. Echo is not playing a character; she *truly believes* that she is a sexy devotee to the cultists' cause. After being fitted with cameras in her retinas, she is the perfect secret agent. For the cult leader, she is irresistibly sexual and a believer. For the government she is a willing participant in national security efforts and the "War on Terror".

In the following dialogue in the same episode of *Dollhouse* a conversation is taking place between Echo's handler, Boyd, and the ATF agents that are monitoring the cult. The dialogue is broken by images of Echo being prepared for the assignment. I have included a brief description of these moments as they intersect the dialogue:

> *Female ATF Agent*: 48 hours to penetrate a closed group? To gain their confidence? To get inside?
> *ATF Agent Lilly*: I'd like you all to meet Boyd Langton. Private contractor recommended to us by Senator Boxbaum. He's been vetted at the highest level. I'll let him tell you what he does.
> *Boyd Langton*: Hi, so, what I do is I work with an extraordinary young woman.
> [broken by images of Echo getting a massage in the Dollhouse]
> *Boyd*: She's not a law enforcement officer. She's not an undercover agent. She's just a girl. She's going to help us.
> [broken by images of Echo being called to the brain programming room of the Dollhouse]
> *Boyd*: Her name is Esther Carpenter, and she knows these people. She knows them like she knows herself.
> *ATF Agent*: What did she escape from a cult?
> *Boyd*: No.
> [broken by images of Echo lying on a table. She has a device over her eyes and there is equipment around. A gloved hand picks up a scalpel]

Boyd: She didn't escape from anything. Esther's talent is not in getting out, but getting in.

[broken by images of a drill heading for Echo's eye]

Boyd: And because of this talent...

[broken by images of a Dollhouse scientist constructing the brain imprint for Echo's assignment]

Boyd: ... because of who she is, that is what she will do. She will not arrive there a stranger or an intruder. She will walk through the gates of the compound and she will be accepted as one of them.

Female ATF Agent: How?

Boyd: Through a miracle.[84]

Certainly, it is a post-9/11 (and perhaps post-Waco, post-Ruby Ridge) miracle. If only the US had a sexually-charge martial arts expert who literally becomes whoever the government needs *in reality*. In an alarming twist, Echo, who is supposed to be playing the blind religious fanatic Esther Carpenter, incorporates part of an earlier mission into her infiltration of the cult. When she is threatened and slapped by the cult leader, Jonas Sparrow, she fights back and ultimately saves the day with a combination of physical violence and heroic courage. Perhaps the only drawback of Echo as an agent of terrorsex is that she has been built and sustained by a greedy corporation with desires of world domination.

The underground corporation that runs the *Dollhouse* forms a powerful post-9/11 metaphor for the military-industrial complex. In his book appropriately titled *The Pornography of Power*, Robert Scheer tracks the gloomy underbelly of post-9/11 government spending and the disturbing links between private corporations and government and military organizations.[85] According to Sheer:

In admitting his difficulty in defining the word "pornography", exasperated Supreme Court Justice Potter Stewart stated, "I know it when I see it". That is how I feel about the use of the word in the title of this book. What it suggests to me is a *vicarious experience that masks the real deal*, substituting lurid and excitable imagery for an activity that is all too mundane and predictable.[86]

It would be difficult to describe the pornography of terror more succinctly. This pornography of power was also a crucial theme in the long-running *The X Files* television series and movies. This program told the stories of FBI Agents Fox Mulder and Dana Scully as they investigated the paranormal and the bizarre. Much of the series focused on a coming alien invasion facilitated by quasi-governmental conspirators in partial collaboration with a mysterious private military corporation called *Roush Technologies*.[87]

Programs like the *X-Files* and *Dollhouse* tap into our fears of government power as much as our fears of being the targets of some kind of terrorist, or perhaps space alien, violence. Following Zillah Eisenstein, all of the figures that I have explored in this chapter – promiscuous women submitting and being forced into body searches for national security, whores and secret agents, and sinister military-industrial corporations – operate as "decoys" in the War on Terror. Decoys can be distracting, they divert our attention, and prevent us from keeping focus in those places where we are most threatened. What better way to distract witnesses from terrorism than by fusing terrorism with sex, *as though terrorism was not already seductive enough.*

Decoys of Terrorsex

Zillah Eisenstein argues that in an age of terror we are surrounded by racialized and gendered "decoys" that work to re-focus our attentions away from the most malignant forms of violence in the US government and military responses to 9/11.[88] She argues that decoys work to re-directed our attentions, re-focus our perspective and allow Western witnesses to tolerate the actions of their governments and militaries that were the willing allies of the US terror war. These decoys are sustained by powerful figures. People such as Condoleeza Rice and Colin Powell work to provide otherwise white, male, heteronormative advice to minorities and marginalized people.

> The wars of/on terror use women and people of color like Colin Powell and Rice as imperial decoys while liberal democratic rights are dismantled at home and nowhere in sight in Afghanistan or Iraq. Arab men are unmanly; and anti-war

activists become girlie men. Imperial democracy has always been defined by sexual and racial conquest. As such this form of democracy has required imperial repression, and now gender(ing) becomes war in yet another form. This war is fought with more females than any previous war while women still also continue to birth the next generation.[89]

But what is this role for women in the terror war? The "War on Terror" is a location for gendered "decoys" where "manly men" and promiscuous women work to ensure our national security.[90] Counterterrorism conferences can be a powerful example of this. These conferences are filled with men, many former and current military personnel, former and current spooks (who sometimes describe themselves in the most cringe-worthy fashion as "trench-coat wearing folk") and government and security bureaucrats. There is the occasional woman, most commonly drawn from more flowery segments of the security and counterterrorism communities – law foundations and organizations, civil rights groups, human services agencies. Even more commonly they are the assistants and secretaries for male counterterrorism big-wigs. In one almost surreal moment from a counterterrorism laws symposium I attended, an increasingly frustrated male security bureaucrat called his female secretary into action during a debate about the definition of terrorism. She handed him a large ring-bound folder opened to a page containing the Australian legislative definition of terrorism. He interrupted the debate, loudly proclaimed the "official" definition of terrorism, snapped the folder shut in an authoritative manner and thrust the folder into the lap of his female secretary. Indeed, counterterrorism conferences can sometimes resemble the anti-female, heteronormative, white-male meccas of male team sports change-rooms. A towel snapping may not have been far away.

For Eisenstein, "In real life, war rages in Afghanistan and Iraq but as a backdrop and not front and center". Meanwhile, terrorsex functions as a powerful decoy in the "War on Terror". Women's roles in this decoying have been made perfectly clear. They are promiscuous national security threats, whores and agents of government counterterrorism efforts, and assistants and secretaries to white-men who make national security work. Eisenstein argues that "Since September 11, 2001 there is a female face to the wars on/ of terror but the meanings of this is not self-evident".[91]

> Females assist in the orchestration of the US wars of/on terror and therefore women have more complicity in these wars than they used to. Yet there is nothing more undemocratic than war so it is highly unlikely that women's presence can mean anything good. No one's rights – especially not women's – can be met in war, or by waging war.[92]

A post-9/11 joke from stand-up comic Margaret Cho sheds a particular light on this problem: "I have been in New York a lot and I actually got a chance to go down to Ground Zero and I was there day after day, giving blowjobs to rescue workers … Yeah. Because we all have to do our part".[93] This followed comments made by Art Spiegelman that he wanted to incorporate into his graphic novel *In the Shadow of No Towers* scenes of "terror sex" in response to the rumors that women were rushing to Ground Zero to "comfort" male rescue workers at night.[94]

The post-9/11 role of women is closely related to the fusion of terrorism and sex that forges *terrorsex*. Here terrorism, war and politics are linked with sex in its commodified form. Perhaps predictably the destruction of the phallic Twin Towers paved the way for a series of identity crises – the destruction of economic power has created a type of masculinized impotence in the face of the catastrophic destruction on 9/11. The commodity of terrorsex should be viewed as an impotent attempt to reclaim lost masculinity and lost power. The age-old myths of naturalized male hegemony is one thing that 9/11 could not change.

Conclusion: The Jenna Jameson Effect

Jenna Massoli was raised in Las Vegas. When she was 18 she changed her name legally to Jenna Jameson. She is now one of the richest pornographic film stars in history. She has starred in over 110 films and is the proprietor of her own website that sells many "Jenna" related products ranging from "bobble head dolls, anatomically correct body parts, mouse pads, vibrators and Zippo lighters".[95] She was the first porn star to become commodified through her image in non-pornographic enterprises when she became the poster girl for *Pony* athletic goods. She once told a reporter that she does not need to work in movies because her image financially sustains her lifestyle: she chooses to work regardless. Jenna Massoli is a person: the commodified image that is Jenna Jameson is dependent on Jenna Massoli. Where Jenna Jameson is the icon of pornographic imagery, 9/11 is the icon of terrorism imagery. Each continued to trade on that image, that spectacle, long after it has been generated. Baudrillard argued that images matter most in their impact and that the difference between "true or false is beside the point".[96]

> We are henceforth – and forever – in a state of uncertainty where images are concerned. Only their impact counts … They no longer represent; they no longer imply either distance or perception or judgement. They are no longer of the order of representation, or of information in the strict sense and, as a result, the question of whether they should be produced, reproduced, broadcast or banned, and even the "essential" question of whether they are true or false, is "irrelevant".[97]

Terrorsex is where representation gives way to excesses: excesses of seeing, excesses of destruction, and excesses of attraction. Predictably, the responses have also been excessive. Invasion and war in the name of 9/11 has claimed far more lives than the terror itself. Yet it could be argued that the response to 9/11 was no more or less proportionate than the reaction to other spectacles. Marilyn Manson tours still attract protests from various segments of the community, as do Eminem's and Snoop Doggy Dogg's tours. The release of the film *American Psycho*, based on the novel about the serial killer Patrick Bateman written by Bret Easton Ellis, also attracted protesters. For some, spectacles spark horror and disgust. For others they are consumable commodities that fulfill fantasies. The spectacle can sometimes be sickly sweet through its paradoxical abhorrence and the excitement it exerts. Its appeal is as predictable as the outcries in opposition.

Pornography generates over two billion dollars a year. Its success as a commodity is difficult to deny. Until recently, the pornography industry relied on the courage of men to visit "seedy stores with no windows and strange lighting and mail orders which were delivered in dubious packaging denoting the obvious".[98] The Internet has not only established a site for pornographic experimentation and image exchange, it has made it more acceptable, routine, banal and everyday. So called soft-core pornography is available in men's entertainment magazines, on television programs, especially "reality" television like *Big Brother* and *Real World*, and in women's magazines promoting fashion. In these conditions, that Baudrillard described as experimental reality, terrorsex has become the commodity of choice.[99] It combines explosions, airplane hijackings, and buildings falling with promiscuity, sexual ambiguity, and pornography. Terrorsex, understood in this way, embodies distinctions between a world of image-events, histories, occurrences and incidents and a world of images, pictures, representations, appearances, illustrations and projections.

The meanings of 9/11 will likely remain contested and it will be reanimated in ever more spaces and sites and in many commodified forms. In the virtual world of "Second Life" for example – a world where communities in different locations coexist in real time in virtual spaces – terrorsex has already taken on new forms. Not only do avatars sexually harass and assault other avatars,[100] but organized groups, such as the *Second Life Liberation Army* (SLLA), engage in virtual terrorist attacks mostly against American owned stores. In an act of virtual disobedience, at a Second Life press conference with a property developer that was hosted "in-world", giant penises scrolled across the virtual environment in what Second Life creator, Philip Rosedale, described as terrorists taking "control of the weather".[101] Perhaps a virtual world has never been so real.

"Who is Jenna Massoli?" and "What is terrorism?" These are two questions that are more difficult to answer than "Who is Jenna Jameson?" and "What is 9/11?" de Plazaola argues that Jameson is the author of her own image that exists independent of her corporeality, but this is not entirely of her own doing.[102] So too does the image – the idea – of 9/11 mean so much more than "terrorism". Jameson has a thriving fan base purchasing her merchandise, visiting her website, and interacting with her in real time online.

As spectators her fans contribute to her image. Witnesses of 9/11 literally embody its meanings, consequences and impacts and give terrorism its power to terrify. 9/11 has a fan base that ensures it will be invoked again and again in reanimating the latest terror scare. As Jenna Jameson has become both a real person and a projected image she is continually animated and reanimated as the projected fantasies of her fan base. The Jameson image is sustained by her sexual appeal and by people being unable to look away. She has continually transformed her image to reflect the demands of the marketplace, her commodified existence, which is her best known existence. This is the Jenna Jameson effect. This is the power of terrorsex.

8.

A Screen Culture of Terrorism

People love fireworks.[1]

It was my sense in the fall of 2001 that the United States was missing an opportunity to redefine itself as part of a global community when, instead, it heightened nationalist discourses, extended surveillance mechanisms, suspended constitutional rights, and developed forms of explicit and implicit censorship.[2]

Talking about 9/11 can be challenging. There have been many occasions when I have been told that I don't take 9/11 seriously enough, that I disrespect the victims by analyzing 9/11 in popular, tele-visual and screen cultures with my academic theories and tricks, that my view from the ivory tower is a distorted one. I have been told that my career should not benefit from 9/11. I have been told that maybe the best thing I can do is be quiet. I have been told that I am standing on the wrong building.

As the quote from Judith Butler that prefaces this conclusion indicates, 9/11 provided an opportunity for some burnt bridges to be mended. It was a moment when many felt a deep and sincere sympathy for the suffering and pain being experienced by all Americans. Yet this opportunity quickly faded as wars were planned, revenge was demanded, and an ill defined enemy was pursued to third world countries which have been decimated as a result. Americans had a right to be sad and angry. But the world's only superpower, capable of destroying the world many times over, needed to show more restraint than it did.

The military response was furious, spectacular and killed many more people and destroyed many more buildings than the 9/11 hijackers. It was, sadly, a hopelessly disproportionate response in a US quest to feel safe again. As Butler writes:

> To be injured means that one has the chance to reflect upon injury, to find out the mechanisms of its distribution, to find out who else suffers from permeable borders, unexpected violence, dispossession, and fear, and in what ways ... the dislocation from First World privilege, however temporary, offers a chance to start to imagine a world in which that violence might be minimized.[3]

Instead, we witnessed operation *shock and awe*. We witnessed the idiocy of "mission accomplished". We continue to witness perpetual war. Some people, perhaps, just love fireworks.

The post-9/11 world is one that is sustained by a failure of imagination. It is a provocation that I direct at all of 9/11's witnesses and a challenge to those grappling with its meanings and consequences. It is a challenge for the always situated witness and the ambiguous and ambivalent "we".

Witnessing Violence

The experience of 9/11 is a story that has been told many times. 9/11 stories, according to Butler, were most characterized by first-person narratives; narratives that personalized 9/11. Where were you? What were you doing? For Butler, the "I" of 9/11 became its universal experience. The "I" captured that "enormous narcissistic wound" that the 9/11 terrorists opened through the "public display of our physical vulnerability".[4] These narratives of "I" – and, perhaps, "we" – are limitless. I want to single out a few in this conclusion.

For blogger and New Yorker "Andy H", 9/11 was a day that started like any other:

On September 11th, 2001 I went to work as usual at the
Woolworth Building, two blocks from the World Trade Center. It was a beautiful day, warm with a clear blue sky. I got
to work around 8:30 a.m., sat down at my desk and turned
on my computer. Then I heard a loud bang.[5]

Andy H was going to work – a routine affair for city-dwellers.
The routine was broken by a "loud bang" and the horror that followed.

Oh, My God!!! THERE'S PEOPLE!!! People jumping out
to escape the flames and falling hundred and hundreds of
feet!!!!!! This is unbearable!!! Shocking. Terrifying.[6]

For Andy H routine gave way to horrific violence. But in these moments after 9/11 began, what can we say that he was witnessing?
In these moments, moments before it had been confirmed as a terrorist attack, Andy was witnessing violence in its most spectacular
and pure form. New York City; a plane accident; death, horror and
destruction. People falling from the sky.

I was watching, we were watching the first WTC building,
watching the people fall and the flames burn when I saw
a plane, a passenger size plane, come out of the sky, arc
around and crash DIRECTLY into the other tower!! It left a
huge hole and smoke and flames. People in the office were
shouting and crying. Someone yelled GET OUT and we
all walked the stairs down to the ground. The streets were
crazy. People wandering around, dazed, crying, freaked out
… I don't know what to say. I really don't. This is beyond
description. Beyond words.[7]

Even after watching a second plane hit the World Trade Center
Andy remained stuck in the images of spectacular violence. When
in the rapture of spectacular terrorism there was no sense of why
this had occurred, no need to know the geopolitical causality, no
wish for revenge, no capacity yet for anger.

So, it's later this afternoon. We've been watching the coverage all morning and afternoon. Phone calling friends. Touching base. Trying to make sure everyone's okay, letting everyone know that I'm okay. It's been an exhausting, emotional day.

I think I'm still in shock.

I can't get the pictures out of my mind: watching people leap to their deaths, choosing between being immolated alive or crushed by falling. I saw one woman, and I know it's impossible, but I could have sworn I heard her scream. It's something you can't imagine. I never thought I could imagine.

Every time I see that footage of that plane hitting the second tower, I twitch.

The thing is that as we looked out the windows of the office, trying to comprehend how a plane could possibly run into the World Trade Center, we just thought it was a horrible, horrible accident. But watching that other plane come in defied belief. And then it just crashed right in. Fire. Smoke. Horror.

There really aren't words.

I can't find the words.

Not now.

Maybe later.

But not now.

Through Andy's words, words of one of 9/11's witnesses, other witnesses (like me) witness 9/11 again and again in different ways. Andy's blog contains only one image of the Towers burning. For the most part it is just words; internet text. But the emotion it conveys is powerful. As I read his blog his words combined with the tele-visual images of 9/11 that I witnessed in the real-time news coverage that are forever stuck in my mind. I can't stop thinking about what he must have experienced, how it must have felt. Our experiences are so different, but we are both witnesses.

Alisa Solomon, writing in *The Village Voice* on 9/11, attempted to capture the emotion of being in New York.[8]

As we trudged along—strangers talking like old friends, people who managed to find cabs and offering to share them—I flashed on the grammar-school drills I went through in the '60s. The Cold War came to my Midwestern suburban school in the form of duck-and-cover exercises and, once a year, a practice evacuation. We were let out of school early and had to walk all the way home, filing out in neat lines and heading into the streets, kids peeling off as we came to their neighborhoods.[9]

Re-animated in this account is the Cold War legacy of fear experienced by many. This was not the first time I had heard a post-9/11 account of those "grammar-school drills" from the 1960s, a time when some believed that the world was at the brink of nuclear annihilation. An American economics lecturer, that taught a class that I was in on 9/11, told us that he hoped that we would not be subject to the same "duck and cover" drills that he had experienced. He feared that the post-9/11 world would make the need for such training essential. Solomon continued:

A real war has come to these shores now, bringing massive violence into America for the first time. The terrible human casualties of today's attacks haven't even begun to be counted yet. Some of the intangible ones to come are obvious—the First Amendment, for starters. The altered city skyline is only the most visible manifestation of the size of the change.[10]

Solomon's account was without the blame, the anger and the thirst for revenge that would come to characterize the weeks and months that followed. She shared her fears for America, for the "First Amendment" and for America's image. The destruction of the Twin Towers proved to be the most "visible manifestation" of the destruction that would be carried out in the name of 9/11.

Toby Miller is a UK-born academic who was at the time of 9/11 living and working in New York City. Toby Miller is deep within the so-called "culture wars" – a prominent member of the academic elite who has, since 9/11, written extensively about American culture and the post-9/11 world. This was his 9/11.

> In bars and elsewhere, I met people with other stories: one guy had been in the subway on the way to work when smoke filled the car. He told me that noone could breathe properly and people were screaming. But his only thought was for his dog DeNiro back in Brooklyn. From the panic of the train, he managed to call his mom on a cell phone to ask her to feed DeNiro that night, because it looked like he wouldn't get home. A pregnant woman told me she had feared for her unborn as she fled the blasts, pushing the pram with her baby in it as she did so. Away from these heart-rending tales from strangers, there was the fear: what horrible price would the US Government extract for this, and who would be the overt and covert agents and targets of that suffering? What blood-lust would this generate? What would be the pattern of retaliation and counter-retaliation? And what would become of domestic civil rights and cultural inclusiveness?[11]

In Miller's account we again witness a fear that extends beyond a fear of international terrorists and their destructive capabilities. A fear of the US's revenge, the curbing of freedoms, and the inevitability of future terrorism as a consequence of these actions. Different witnesses, different stories – yet these stories are so similar. They are stories of witnessing – in one way or another – an incredible event, an event so violent, an event so unlike any others that have occurred in cities during times of peace.

> The sounds of lower Manhattan that used to serve as white noise for residents – sirens, screeches, screams – were no longer signs without a referent. Instead, they made folks stare and stop, hurry and hustle, wondering whether the noises we thought we knew so well were coefficients of a new reality. In the intervening months, the US media and war planners have supplied their own narrow frameworks, making New York's "ground zero" into the starting point

for escalating global violence. There has been no reflexivity whatsoever about the history of US aggression or militarism, its policies of attrition and destruction in the Third World and its internal plutocratic workings. How could this be?[12]

Violence of the scale of 9/11 is a daily occurrence in some parts of the world. Some people live in perpetual war. I wonder what 3000 dead means to someone living and working in Brazzaville, Congo (one of the world's most violent cities) or perhaps Baghdad? Certainly, 3000 dead is a huge number for people living in the developed or even the developing world. For these people 9/11 is – in more ways than one – *a new referent*. It is a new referent for violence, for cosmopolitan city living, for all terrorism past and present, for all post-9/11 terror scares, and, importantly for this book, for diverse fields in popular, tele-visual and screen cultures.

The creators, writers and directors of these cultures were witnesses too even if they communicated their witnessing in ways that are different to western academics, bloggers, or magazine journalists. I have shared their witnessing – their 9/11s – throughout this book. They have shown us what they witnessed through their films and television programs, with the characters they created, with the post-9/11 storylines they shared. Their witnessing, it seems, was not only about 9/11. It was about so much more. It was about dealing with trauma and living with the meanings and consequences of 9/11. It was about dwelling in a world that is indefinitely described as post-9/11. It is a world where "9/12" was the first day of the rest of our lives.

9/12

Eliot Weinberger writes of what it felt like to be living in New York City on 12 September 2001; what he calls in the title of his book "9/12"[13]:

It is, of course, impossible to know what the effects of yesterday's horror will be; whether it will permanently alter the national psyche (if there is one) or merely recede as yet another bundle of images from yet another media spectacle.

This is clearly the first event since the rise of the omnipotence of mass media that is larger than the media, that the media cannot easily *absorb and tame*. If the media do succeed, national life, beyond the personal tragedies, will continue in its semi-hallucinatory state of continual manufactured imagery. If they fail, something profound may indeed change.[14]

Did the media succeed or fail in *absorbing and taming* 9/11? Or, could we not equally ask, did 9/11 succeed or fail in absorbing and taming the media and its audiences of witnesses?

Noam Chomsky once argued that underpinning devastating global violence was a "Culture of Terrorism".[15] This culture was a product of US war-making throughout many parts of the world and the propaganda campaign produced and waged by the government's willing allies in the media, academic, political, social and cultural industries. Chomsky has spent the best parts of his career showing that beneath outbursts of violence targeting the US lies a culture of violence, a culture of terrorism, sustained by the US military and their client governments. This global violence proceeded mostly unchallenged with a little help from a complacent media and a population whose *consent* has been *manufactured* through mass-mediated propaganda.[16]

After 9/11, Chomsky continued his quest to articulate the seedy US connections to third world oppression, practices of torture, fascism and illegitimate governments. But 9/11 occurred in a world that was very different to the one in which *The Culture of Terrorism* was penned, a world dominated by wars both hot and cold. Chomsky's belief that people needed to become more informed, less reliant on formalized education and the mass media – dominated as it is by an elite few – was more problematic in a post-9/11 world. It was more problematic on 9/12. Chomsky's notions of the culture of terrorism have been forced to evolve with the hyper-mediated age in which 9/11 continually takes place in popular, tele-visual and screen cultures. There was, after all, few terrorism blogs before 9/11. Tele-vision and film still featured terrorism storylines, but they were not of the same order. Pre-9/11 storylines were more likely to feature Cold War enemies and brave Muslim nationalists than they were to feature anti-Western Islamic radicals. Certainly Seth MacFarlane was not making jokes about terrorism, nor was Matt Stone and Trey Parker highlighting the absurdities of how people respond to terrorism. *Battlestar Galactica* still existed, but in a form barely recognizable to aficionados of the re-imagined BSG. It seems clear that a culture of terrorism still exists, but it exists in a different form. It is a form with many of the hallmarks of Chomsky's analysis (US aggression, third world blow back, a largely compromised mass media). These hallmarks are featured in some of our most viewed screen cultures, and because of this they are unavoidable. No amount of self-induced ignorance will remain blissful for long. This is the contemporary *screen culture of terrorism*.

The Taming Event

The media did not *absorb and tame* 9/11, it is 9/11 that has tamed the media, screen cultures and their audiences. Did camera operators choose where they should point their cameras on 9/11, or was this decision already made? 9/11 made this decision on behalf of all cameras, camera operators, media producers, creators and – most importantly – media consumers; the global audiences of witnesses that have been the subject of this book. They could not help but watch. They could not look away.

Did 9/11 not *absorb and tame* us all? Has not the post-9/11 world been so absorbed by 9/11 that it now appears in the most routine and mundane ways in our popular, tele-visual and screen cultures? Weinberger argues that before 9/11 the world's media audiences had been so assaulted by overwhelming and violent images in film, television and news media that when 9/11 occurred witnesses had already been desensitized to the images of horror and violence. It reminded him of the "Romans [who] had to pour fish emulsion on their food to bring some taste to palates deadened by the lead in their water pipes".[17]

> Violence had become grotesque, comedies depend on increasingly scatological stupidities which are mistaken for transgressions, adventure films have abandoned narrative to become theme parks offering a special effects thrill a second, corporations manufacture revolutionary rappers

or angry white-boy rock groups, television turns the death
of vaguely remembered celebrities into national days of
mourning and the forecast of routine storms into dire warnings of potential disaster.[18]

What the pre-9/11 world lacked, according to Weinberger, was a
sense of *reality*. But a passion for the real remained. When the real
event occurred – the immeasurable horror of 9/11 – witnesses did
not know what to do with it. Despite being desensitized, witnesses
were horrified, disgusted, appalled. Yet, 9/11 was still dealt with by
incorporating it into the banal and routine narratives of post-9/11
life. It was, perhaps, the only way that we could survive. By bury-
ing the reality of 9/11 in banal routines we disavowed the violence,
and in the process we "rediscover[ed]" daily life.[19]

This was how 9/11 found its way so easily into popular, tele-visual and screen cultures. This was how the television show *Friends*
so quickly and subtly changed. This was how shows like *How I Met
Your Mother* were born (a show that is somehow about 9/11, yet in
no way incorporates 9/11 into the story; we simply accept that it is
there). This was how the infamous seventies cult classic *Battlestar
Galactica* was reborn in ways not unlike the humanoid Cylons themselves – death marked a re-birth. This was how comedy could be so
blended with trauma. This was how a photographer for *Vogue: Italia*
thought it would be arousing if his latest sexualized fashion shoot
took place in a counterterrorism context. For Baudrillard this is the
"spectacle of banality"; "the obscene spectacle of nullity, insignificance and platitude".[20] It was also how we returned to our lives.

This is perhaps why television shows like *Friends* proceeded
as normal after 9/11, as though nothing had happened, as though
nothing had changed. When I presented a paper on this subject at
a national conference on sociology in Australia I was confronted as
I was leaving the stage by a woman, an academic working in Australia at the time, who identified herself as a New Yorker. She was
angry, even furious. Her voice was quivering as she snapped at me
that I did not know what I was talking about and that people like
me had no right to talk about 9/11. I was immediately concerned
that I had said something off-the-cuff that had made light of the
tragedy of 9/11 and I quickly replayed my talk in my head search-

ing for my transgression. Finding nothing I asked her what she meant, she simply replied that I had no right, *I was not a New Yorker*. I was concerned that I had upset this New Yorker, but I could not help but ponder her aggressive response to what I considered to be a fairly routine paper about how 9/11 had been represented in a popular television show. My thoughts following this confrontation became an impetus for this book. I questioned myself constantly. Had I shed light on the silence and absence of 9/11 in Friends, or was I being insulting, playing down the significance of the attack? Had I, by highlighting the everydayness of 9/11, intruded on her long and hard recovery from 9/11?

What I came to believe were some of the answers to this question can, once again, be articulated through tele-visual allegory. This allegory comes from a familiar place; Matt Stone and Trey Parker and their *South Park* television series.

Terrorists Have Attacked Our Imaginations, and Our Imaginations Have Run Wild

The eleventh season of *South Park* featured a trilogy of episodes that focused on the meanings and consequences of terrorism. These episodes were named "Imaginationland" episodes I, II and III.[21] In this trilogy audiences witness a peculiar story of a major act of terror that has devastating consequences for witnesses throughout the world. This act of terror did not occur in a major city, at an airport, in a tall building or on the public transport network. Indeed, the terrorists in these *South Park* episodes had learnt to by-pass these locations and deploy a more direct strategy. They attacked our imaginations. Or, to be more precise, a fantastic and magical place known as *Imaginationland*.

The first episode in the trilogy began with Eric Cartman attempting to convince his friends that he had seen a Leprechaun. With some maintaining their disbelief, Cartman set out to capture the Leprechaun. Ultimately, he failed, but Cartman and the other South Park children learn that the Leprechaun was rushing back to Imaginationland to warn of an impending terrorist attack. He feared that he was too late. Whilst waiting for the school bus the following morning, the children encountered a strange old man dressed in strange clothes and a top hat. He was searching for the

Leprechaun. When the children told him that they had encountered the Leprechaun he invited them back to his home as his guests. He was the Mayor of Imaginationland. The children climbed aboard his enchanted sky-ship (which looks like an 18th century explorer's boat) and they made the journey to Imaginationland. Shortly after they arrived, a shriek is heard and cartoon versions of suicide bombers storm into Imaginationland and detonate their bomb-vests.

Viewers witness the cartoon carnage of the aftermath of these attacks. We witness visual horrors that include Ragedy Anne nursing the mangled, life-less body of Ragedy Andy; a burning Santa Claus accidently setting on fire those who try to help him; Ronald McDonald, missing one arm, searching for, and finding, his missing limb; and streets littered with the corpses of unicorns, Smurfs and other fictional creatures. We see other terrorists open fire with machine guns. The terrorists are comedic and exaggerated characters designed to appeal to western stereotypes of what an Islamic extremist looks like. *South Park* is a crudely drawn cartoon, but the images of a terrorist attack on Imaginationland manage to be grotesque and disturbing. The children escaped on the back of a dragon and returned to the *real* world to report the attack to the US government. They woke up in their beds, thinking that they had been dreaming, only to discover that they all had the same dream and that their friend, Butters, was missing, left behind in Imaginationland.

Keyes argues that the allegory of a terrorist attack directly targeting our imaginations "suggests America's foreign policy may be more about a failure of the imagination than a failure to properly export American cultural dominance".[22] Indeed, this "failure" of foreign policy is captured through ironic conversations that take place between the government and military officials in the Imaginationland episodes. In the following scene we witness one such conversation as they prepared their counterterrorism responses to the attack on Imaginationland. This conversation proceeded on the basis that a terrorist attack had literally occurred. The impossibility, intangibility, ambiguity and ambivalence of the terrorists' imaginary targets was never questioned. The fact that our imaginations is a place that is not of the same order as New York City or London is never part of the equation. For these cartooned military and government counterterrorism officials, Imaginationland might as well be a geographical location in continental USA.

> *General*: Ladies and gentlemen, I have dire news. Yesterday, at approximately 18:00 hours, terrorists successfully attacked [pause for effect] our imagination.
> *Government official 1*: Our imagination?
> *Government official 2*: How?
> *CT Specialist*: The imaginary attack appears to have been in the works for years. The effects of the attack are so far unimaginable.
> *General*: … Luckily we've kept it from being broadcast to the public … Gentlemen, the terrorists appear to have complete control of our imagination. It's only a matter of time before our *imaginations start running wild*.[23]

In their analysis of the Imaginationland trilogy, Sienkiewicz and Marx focus on the representations of Muslim terrorists.[24] The authors argue that the terrorists that attacked Imaginationland were themselves "exaggerated and buffoonish caricatures" leading to the inevitable question "what do Muslim terrorists have to do with mermaids and Mighty Mouse?"[25] Representations of Muslims in popular, tele-visual and screen cultures have quite a bit in common with other fictional characters. Popular images of Muslims such as the ones in the Imaginationland trilogy are themselves *fictional* – they are more indicative of how Muslim terrorists are stereotyped, not how they might appear in a police line-up. This was clearly one of Stone and Parker's goals; to demonstrate how the "War on Terror" works to privilege imaginary image-realities over everyday realities. The imaginary Muslim was held in sharp focus throughout the Imaginationland episodes. In the following scene, the government and military officials are viewing a video that they had received from the Imaginationland terrorists:

> [*on the video*] *Mayor of Imaginationland*: No! It's just a Care Bear!
> [*watching the video*] *Government official*: Oh my God!

> [*watching the video*] General: Later in the video we can see another imaginary hostage; this one reading a forced statement.
>
> [*on the video*] Butters: Praise to the mighty Allah. His divine grace and will have brought forth this day. [*a terrorist brings forth the severed head of a Care Bear and holds it in front of the camera*] Oh jeez! Uhhh, n..now see, your safety is at our whim. This is the price you pay, America! You have defiled Allah, and now we will turn your imagination against you! Death to the Infidels![26]

In this scene we witness a recreation of a fearsome post-9/11 moment – a terrorists' captive being beheaded on television. Several videos of beheadings are available on the internet. Television networks decided not to show these videos on their broadcasts. I have had the misfortune of witnessing one of these videos myself. I believed it was part of my job as a terrorism studies academic. I felt that hiding myself from the actions of terrorists would mean that I was failing in my duties. I don't plan to witness one again. They are sickening. For this reason I found this scene in *South Park* to be a little distasteful. This was, of course, the point. I found it distasteful because it was already in my imagination. If I had not been exposed to the post-9/11 world, then the beheading of a Care Bear would be unlikely to cause offense. But, naturally, the beheading of the Care Bear was designed as a symbolic act. It demonstrates how 9/11 and the subsequent terror war has captured our imaginations. My offense demonstrates that the terrorist attack on my imagination has been a successful one.

Keyes argues that the Imaginationland episodes demonstrate that our greatest fears may well lie "deep inside the entertainment industry's image gallery".[27] It should not be surprising that Hollywood directors M. Night Shyamalan and Michael Bay were called to help in preparing a counterterrorism response to the attacks on Imaginationland:

> General: What I am about to tell you is highly classified. Two days ago, Muslim terrorists hijacked our imagination. Frankly we don't know what their next move is or how to stop them.

CT Specialist: In times like these the government often turns to Hollywood for help. You creative filmmakers can think of ideas we just can't.

General: That's why we've asked you here, M. Night Shyalamalam. *The Sixth Sense, Signs, The Village*, all very clever films. But can you use your amazing idea brain now to help us stop the terrorists?

M. Night Shyamalan: What if ... What if it turns out they aren't terrorists? But they're actually werewolves? From the future?

General: N, no. No, they're terrorists. They've been linked to Al Qaeda.

M. Night Shyamalan: But what if Al Qaeda, it turns out, is the group being terrorized? By aliens?

General: No- No. That's not an idea, that's a twist. We need ideas.

M. Night Shyalaman: How about we make everyone think that terrorists attacked us? But really, we were all already dead.

General: Get him out of here.

General: Mr. Bay, can you think of any idea how to outwit these terrorists?

Michael Bay: I believe I can. We start by making a big CG [computer generated] building and then we have a meteor go CROSSHH! and it, and it's all like CRAAWWW a-and motorcycles burst into flame while they jump over these helicopters, right?

General: No no! We need ideas how to stop the terrorists!

Michael Bay: An eighteen-wheeler spins out of control and it's all like CROSSHH and then this huuuge tanker full of dyna- CROSSH BRAAWWW

General: Those aren't ideas, those are special effects!

Michael Bay: [long pause] I... don't understand the difference.

General: I know you don't. Get him out of here![28]

Pop-culture creators have undoubtedly played a central role in framing the post-9/11 world. As Baudrillard and Žižek have pointed out, they also played a central role in contextualizing the pre-9/11 world and in preparing witnesses for real, catastrophic events.[29] Parker and Stone's provocation that Hollywood directors should play a role in counterterrorism is more serious and pragmatic than it first appears. In the study of terrorism, popular, tele-visual and screen cultures need to be taken seriously. These cultures contextualize our world, our lives. The cultural impact of television programs like *Friends, Battlestar Galactica, The Simpsons, Family Guy* and *South Park* will not be soon forgotten. In many ways, these programs were enlisted to help witnesses respond to terrorism. They are an important part of witnesses' counterterrorism efforts. They have helped us control, organize and sometimes restrain our imaginations. Programs like *Friends, Sex and the City* and *How I Met Your Mother* reminded witnesses that life continues after 9/11 and that people can expect to be happy in the post-9/11 world. The re-imagined BSG and Seth MacFarlane's cultural critiques have helped remind witnesses that it is okay to have doubts, it is okay to be critical, even cynical, and it is okay to become politically frustrated and desire change. Matt Stone and Trey Parker have reminded witnesses that it is okay to laugh at the consequences of terrorism. Engaging popular, tele-visual and screen cultures may be our best hope in preventing our imaginations from running wild.

Assuming the Worst – Letting Our Imaginations Run Wild

There is an alarming capacity in the post-9/11 world for witnesses to believe, and assume, the worst. According to Lee Ben Clarke:

> People are worried, now, about terror and catastrophe in ways that a short time ago would have seemed merely fantastic. Not to say that horror and fear suffuse the culture, but they are in the ascendant. And for good reason. There are possibilities for accident and attack, disease and disaster that would make September 11 look like a mosquito bite ... The idea of worst cases isn't foreign to us.[30]

Views such as this – views I am sad to say find sympathetic ears amongst some in the terrorism and counterterrorism extended communities mainly amongst those "experts" with a product to sell – is the equivalent of being a terrorism germ-o-phobe. Parasitic germs are real, and can cause us harm. But given some simple efforts towards cleanliness, they almost certainly will not. Similarly, it is theoretically possible that terrorists could master nuclear weapons, biological agents and methods for chemical, radiological and germ warfare (despite most states not possessing these skills), but I am going to go ahead and believe that they will not. Perhaps this can be the theme of the next Tom Clancy or Stephen King novel. It is farcical to suggest that worst case scenarios should be considered in everyday situations. Clearly, they should not be. Humans have long known that dwelling on worst case scenarios gets us nowhere. In everyday life we hold all manner of risks and threats at arm's length – if we did not do this, we might decide that the most mundane activities, such as driving our cars, are too dangerous (perhaps the most statistically dangerous act undertaken by millions of city-dwellers each day). After 9/11, many Americans decided catching planes was too dangerous. They decided to drive instead of flying. Gerd Gigerenzer calculated that in the year following 9/11 there were 1595 deaths as a direct result of people driving instead of flying.[31]

As Clarke acknowledges 9/11 "imprint[ed] upon our imaginations scenes of horror that until then had been the province of novels and movies. We now imagine ourselves in those images, and our wide-awake nightmares are worse than they used to be".[32] Clarke's sound reasoning gives way to a counter-intuitive claim that "warnings that the worst is at hand should be inspected closely".[33] I disagree. A little bit of distance provides perspective and we realize that the threat and consequences of terrorism can be minimal if only we were not so vulnerable to our "wide-awake nightmares". If only our imaginations did not run wild.

I know, however, that it is not this simple. Terrorism is designed so that people will overreact. Terrorists want a lot of people watching, not just a lot of people dead. Acts of terror attract witnesses – this is the terrorists' goal. Terrorism will likely always be a successful tactic to this end. This is not about an overreaction. The suggestion that we are simply overreacting to terrorism is too reductive, although it is part of the story. It is more likely that our reactions are appropriate given 9/11's regular reanimation and symbolic power. 9/11 failed to vanish after it occurred; it lingered, powerfully and spectacularly in acts of terror and terror scares, and in international wars. It has also lingered in screen cultures, reanimated as some of our favorite television shows, films and blogs. I hope that I have demonstrated this throughout this book.

More than anything else, the Imaginationland episodes helped me realize that, surely, I was not being insulting or disrespectful the day that I was confronted by that New Yorker. I came to understand that we were experiencing a difference in witnessing, a difference in *imagining 9/11* and we were equally grappling with 9/11's failure to disappear. Her 9/11 was disrupted by my witnessing, and my 9/11 was disrupted by hers. Perhaps Matt Stone and Trey Parker's 9/11 also disrupts her 9/11, but it does not disrupt my own in the same way. But we – this New Yorker and I – are not without commonalities. *We* were (and are) witnesses of 9/11 and the parade of post-9/11 images and events that it generated. In this respect we are kin in "Imaginationland".

An Undifferentiated We

When I talked about "we" in this book I did intend, in many respects, for it to be understood as an undifferentiated "we" – a "we" that homogenizes, unifies and brings together people with diverse cultural, social, political, gendered, classed and socio-economic backgrounds. This was, in a very real sense, the level at which the 9/11 terrorists *pitched* their attacks – as a global image-event. In other respects, this undifferentiated "we" is problematic and, indeed, must be problematized. The witnessing that "we" engaged in on and after 9/11 is radically different across multiple configurations of time and space. In short, there is different witnessing. I may have witnessed these attacks differently to everybody else. There are times when I cannot even be certain that what I am witnessing in popular, tele-visual and screen cultures is really there – if it is *really real*.

Yet, I refuse to believe that I am alone in my witnessing. More than this, I still believe that even some, possibly many, New Yorkers share my witnessing as well. As the New Yorker Eliot Weinberger argues:

> Of the many indelible images of the Trade Center attack, the one that I think, or hope, will have a permanent effect is that of the plane crashing into the tower. It was immediately perceived by everyone – it couldn't help but be – as a scene from a movie, one that even, by the second day, became available in different camera angles. America, as it has often been said, has become the place where the unreality of the media is the reigning reality, where everyday life is the self-conscious, ironic parody of what is seen on the various screens. But what will it mean when the realization sinks in that this ultimate simulacrum, the greatest special effect ever, led to the very real death of people one knows and the destruction of a place where one once stood?[34]

This collective act of witnessing is shared by millions of people throughout the world. Some witnessed in real-time as the events were occurring; some witnessed the shocking and obscene wars waged in 9/11's name; some witnessed the popular, tele-visual and screen cultural representations. Indeed, 9/11 touched many lives in differing and sometimes surprising ways. It was, without a doubt, an attack on our cities, our friends, families, colleagues and kin, and an attack on our imaginations.

This attack on our imaginations – an attack waged by both terrorists and counterterrorists – mixes with the power of spectacular images to create a potent concoction where images and violence combine to create something more powerful than images or violence alone. These images are seductive, and as witnesses we are compelled to watch. When framed in this way, we can learn much about our response to 9/11 from Julia Kristeva's work on the imaginary and the spectacle. As a follower of Guy Debord's notions of the "society of the spectacle"[35], a society where spectacular and glistening media surfaces come to define relations between people, Kristeva argues that our fantasies are impoverished since they are transplanted from our imaginations to ubiquitous screen cultures.[36] Out capacity to imagine bows to the hyperreality of the image – an image that defines the criteria by which reality comes to be located and fixed. Because of this, as post-9/11 witnesses we are no longer in control of anything that could be considered an *imaginary self*. We experience a disconnection from our image-reality – we can define what we are seeing, but we (contrary to Lee Ben Clarke's claim) struggle to put ourselves in the picture.[37] The trauma that this displacement causes forces witnesses to spin out what Žižek calls "intricate symbolic cobwebs" – symbolic everyday realities.[38] These realities have taken the form of popular, tele-visual and screen cultures that represent what we think we have seen and what we think it means.

> This empire of the spectacle ... leads to what I have called, "new maladies of the soul": our capacity to represent conflicts within ourselves; to be free and to rebel, to have an interior life – that is, a "soul", a "psyche" – is threatened. The imaginary is standardised ... What can be done? We can work with and against images to develop the kind of imagination that does not stifle the passions, but sublimates them.[39]

What this would mean in practice is a reversal of 9/11's ability to absorb and tame its witnesses. Witnesses must do just as Weinberger hoped – *we must absorb and tame 9/11*. Perhaps if we had achieved this in the immediate aftermath of 9/11 international wars that will produce several generations of terrorists would not have been so hastily waged; war and violence would not have become our daily news-media diet; and perhaps witnesses throughout the world would not fear 9/11's second coming as terrorists (both real and imaginary) continue to threaten our everyday lives. If we absorb and tame 9/11 we will be resilient. If terrorism fails to cause terror there will be nothing to fear.

A Catharsis?

> The city was eerily beautiful last night: silent, sombre, introspective.[40]

Alan Wolfe argues that the two most significant terrorist attacks to have occurred in the US are allegory for the dilemmas faced by terrorism's witnesses as we face the second decade of the twenty-first century. One attack was in Oklahoma City in 1995 – a conservative state, a red state, a state that "symbolizes the side in the culture war that stands for a return to the religion, values, and morality of years past".[41] The other was in Lower Manhattan on 9/11; "probably the most liberal slice of America, represents modern urbane cosmopolitanism, racial and ethnic diversity, and openness to the rest of the world". These attacks bridged political gaps and partisanships, yet, after some time, were the basis for building more walls and more partisan politics.

9/11 has had significant meanings and consequences for people in all parts of the world, even if I have met only a few of them or encountered them as producers and creators of post-9/11 popular, tele-visual and screen cultures. Some witnesses spoke to me about their everyday lives in the vulnerable and precarious city. Some unknowingly spoke to me through the blogosphere. Some made a quirky fictitious manual about being an agent in the fictional "Counterterrorism Unit" on 24 not knowing that I would consider it an essential part of the arguments I make in this book. Some wrote, created and produced television shows. Some re-imagined television shows that already existed. Some honored the victims of 9/11. Some made jokes. Some took photos of partially-dressed models holding guns or stripping at security check points. Some turned secret agents into whores and counterterrorists.

But given all of this, what has 9/11 meant and what will it continue to mean to global audiences of witnesses located in New York and cities and towns throughout the world? Have *we* changed? Has 9/11 sparked some sort of catharsis? *We* still vicariously support war perpetrated by our governments throughout the world, *we* live in ridiculous wealth while others don't have enough food. We rally around political movements that improve our lots in life and advance our interests. Left and right. Conservative and progressive. It is not for me to say definitively who "we" are. That is a decision we all have to make for ourselves.

Perhaps I am part of the problem. Perhaps I offer vicarious support to my government which also waged war against those who were labeled "terrorists" when they fought back. Perhaps I am worse. I am, after all, an academic at a government funded University – I am surely no friend to oppressed people despite any good intentions I might have. Yet if the New Yorker who confronted me is any indication, people like me are not friends to those who are the victims of terrorism either. I have been told that I have made light of their suffering by writing a book about how 9/11 has been represented in screen cultures. Might I be one of the "Little Eichmans" that Ward Churchill referred to? I think I would rather not know.

Having said all of this, my confessions have meant nothing. I don't intend to stop being an academic, nor do I intend to stop writing about 9/11 and terrorism. For me, there is no catharsis. Part of me loves watching television. Watching television after 9/11 makes me feel human, it makes me feel real. This realness allows me to mourn the victims of 9/11 and the victims of the violent reprisals in the so-called "War on Terror". I also mourn those who feel that terrorism is their only option, and those who feel that being a soldier is theirs. But no catharsis does not mean that there is no hope. I have witnessed change in America and the world and I can only hope for a better world for everyone, filled with television and film storylines that don't haunt us with trauma nor condemn us to ignorance.

Notes

Chapter 1

1. Chris Carter and Frank Spotnitz (writers), *The X Files: Fight the Future* (Los Angeles: Twentieth Century Fox, 1998).

2. Luke Howie, *Terrorism, the Worker and the City: Simulations and Security in a Time of Terror* (Surrey, UK: Gower/Ashgate, 2009), 5.

3. Walter Laqueur, *The Age of Terrorism* (Boston: Little, Brown and Company, 1987), 174.

4. Ibid.

5. Ibid.

6. John Tulloch, *One Day in July: Experiencing 7/7* (London: Little, Brown, 2006), 129.

7. Emphasis in original. Zygmunt Bauman, *Does Ethics Have a Chance in a World of Consumers?* (Cambridge: Harvard University Press, 2008), 1.

8. Brian Jenkins, "The Future Course of International Terrorism", in Paul Wilkinson and Alasdair Stewart (eds), *Contemporary Research on Terrorism*, (Aberdeen: Aberdeen University Press, 1987).

9. Donna Haraway, *Modest_Witness@Second_Millenium.FemaleMan©_Meets_OncoMouse™: Feminism and Technoscience* (New York: Routledge, 1997), 267.

10. Ibid.

11. Ibid, 268.

12. Ibid.

13. Ibid, 269.

14. Donna Haraway (interviewed by Thyrza Nichols Goodeve), *How Like a Leaf: An Interview with Thyrza Nichols Goodeve* (New York: Routledge, 2000), 107

15. Donna Haraway, *Simians, Cyborgs and Women: The Reinvention of Nature* (London: Free Association, 1991), 188.

16. Ibid.

17. Ibid, 188-189.

18. Ibid, 189.

19. John Urry, *Mobilities* (Cambridge, UK: Polity, 2007), 143.

20. David Rapoport, "The Four Waves of Modern Terrorism", in Dipak K. Gupta, *Terrorism and Homeland Security* (Belmont: Thomson Wadsworth, 2006); Walter Laqueur, *The New Terrorism: Fanaticism and the Arms of Mass Destruction* (London: Phoenix Press, 1999); Walter Laqueur, *No End to War: Terrorism in the Twenty-First Century* (New York: Continuum, 2003).

21. Walter Laqueur, *No End to War*, 3.

22. Ibid.

23. Ibid, 11.

24. In David Rapoport, "Fear and Trembling: Terrorism in Three Religious Traditions", *American Political Science Review*, 1984, 78 (3), 670.

25. Baljit Singh, "An Overview", in Yonah Alexander and Seymour Finger (eds.), *Terrorism: Interdisciplinary Perspectives* (New York: John Jay Press, 1977), 6, 14; Walter Laqueur, *The New Terrorism*, 11.

26. Baljit Singh, "An Overview", 6, 14; Walter Laqueur, *The New Terrorism*, 11.

27. David Rapoport, "Fear and Trembling", 665.

28. Baljit Singh, "An Overview", 6, 14; Walter Laqueur, *The New Terrorism*, 11.

29. David Rapoport, "Fear and Trembling", 661.

30. Ibid, 660.

31. Ibid; J. Sleeman, *Thugs; Or a Million Murders* (London: S. Low and Marston, 1933).

32. David Rapoport, "Fear and Trembling", 660.

33. Leonard Weinberg, Ami Pedahzur and Sivan Hirsch-Hoefler, "The Challenges of Conceptualizing Terrorism", *Terrorism and Political Violence*, 2004, 16(4).

34. Alex Schmid and A.J. Jongman, *Political Terrorism: A New Guide to Actors, Authors, Concepts, Data Bases, Theories and Literature* (North Holland: Oxford, 1988).

35. Louise Richardson, *What Terrorist's Want: Understanding the Terrorist Threat* (London: John Murray, 2006).

36. See also Jordan J. Paust, "A Definitional Focus", in Yonah Alexander and Seymour Finger (eds.), *Terrorism: Interdisciplinary Perspectives* (New York: John Jay Press, 1977), 18-19; William Waugh, Jr., *International Terrorism: How Nations Respond to Terrorists* (Salisbury: Documentary Publications, 1982), 27; William Waugh, Jr., *Terrorism and Emergency Management* (New York: Marcel Dekker Inc., 1990), 43-49.

37. Louise Richardson, *What Terrorist's Want*, 20.

38. Ibid, 21.

39. Ibid.

40. John Horgan, *The Psychology of Terrorism* (London: Routledge, 2005), 3.

41. Nehemia Friedland and Ariel Merari, "The Psychological Impact of Terrorism: A Double-edged Sword", *Political Psychology*, 1985, 6(4).

42. Slavoj Žižek, *Welcome to the Desert of the Real!: Five Essays on September 11 and Related Dates* (London: Verso, 2002), 11.

43. Gabriel Weimann and Conrad Winn, *The Theatre of Terrorism: Mass Media and International Terrorism* (New York: Longman, 1994).

44. Walter Laqueur, *The New Terrorism*, 12.

45. David Rapoport, "The Four Waves of Modern Terrorism; E. Rauchway, "The President and the Assassin", *The Boston Globe*, 7 September 2003, available at http://www.boston.com/news/globe/ideas/articles/2003/09/07/the_president_and_the_assassin/, retrieved on 15 April 2005.

46. Rick Berg, "Losing Vietnam: Covering the War in an Age of Technology", *Cultural Critique*, 1986, 3, Spring.

47. Ibid, 96.

48. Jack Lule, "Sacrifice and the Body on the Tarmac: Symbolic Significance of U.S News About a Terrorist Victim", in Yonah Alexander and Robert Picard (eds.), *In the Camera's Eye: News Coverage of Terrorist Events* (Washington: Brassey's, 1991), 30.

49. In Barry Rosen, "The Media Dilemma and Terrorism", in Yonah Alexander and Richard Latter (eds.), *Terrorism & the Media: Dilemmas for Government, Journalists & the Public* (Washington: Brassey's, 1990), 58.

50. Emphasis in original. Tom Wicker in Ibid, 58.

51. Tony Atwater, "Network Evening News Coverage of the TWA Hostage Crisis", in Yonah Alexander and Richard Latter (eds.), *Terrorism & the Media: Dilemmas for Government, Journalists & the Public* (Washington: Brassey's, 1990), 88.

52. Jean Baudrillard, *The Spirit of Terrorism and Requiem for the Twin Towers* (London: Verso, 2002), 4.

53. Brigitte Nacos, *Mass-Mediated Terrorism: The Central Role of the Media in Terrorism and Counterterrorism* (Lanham: Rowman and Littlefield Publishers, 2002), 34.

54. Michael Barnett, "From Me to We ... and Back Again: Returning to Business as Usual", *Journal of Management Inquiry*, 2002, 11(3), 249.

55. Toby Miller, "On Being Ignorant: Living in Manhattan", 2002, available at www.portalcomunicacion.com/bcn2002/n_eng/contents/11/miller.pdf, retrieved on 1 February 2007.

56. Kristiaan Versluys, *Out of the Blue: September 11 and the Novel* (New York: Columbia University Press, 2009).

57. Stephen Prince, *Firestorm: American Film in the Age of Terrorism* (New York: Columbia University Press, 2009).

58. Jeffrey Melnick, *9/11 Culture: America Under Construction* (Malden, MA: John Wiley & Sons, 2009).

59. John Law, *After Method: Mess In Social Science Research* (London: Routledge, 2004), 1.

60. Ibid, 13.

61. Ibid.

62. Donna Haraway, *Modest Witness*, 24.

63. Ibid.

64. Ibid, 269.

65. John Law, *After Method*, 24.

66. Ibid, 25.

67. My emphasis. Noam Chomsky (interviewed by Dimitriadis Epaminondas), "On the War Against Terrorism and Related Issues", 3 July 2002, available at http://www.chomsky.info/interviews/20020703.htm, retrieved on 30 March 2008.

68. Peter Manning, *Us and Them: A Journalist's Investigation of Media, Muslims and the Middle East* (Milsons Point, NSW: Random House Australia, 2006).

69. Jean Baudrillard, *The Spirit of Terrorism*, 4.

70. My thanks to Dr. Chris Gellar at Deakin University.

71. Douglas Kellner, *Media Spectacle and the Crisis of Democracy: Terrorism, War and Election Battles* (London: Paradigm, 2005); Henry Giroux, *Beyond the Spectacle of Terrorism: Global Uncertainty and the Challenge of the New Media* (Boulder: Paradigm, 2006).

72. Developed from Luke Howie, *Terrorism, the Worker and the City*, 5.

73. Robert Cochran and Joel Surnow (creators), *24* (Beverly Hills, CA: Imagine Entertainment, 2001).

74. J. J. Abrams (creator), *Alias* (Burbank, CA: Touchstone Television, 2001).

75. Paul Greengrass (writer and creator), *United 93* (Universal City, CA: Universal Pictures, 2006).

76. Andrea Burloff and John McLoughlin (writers), *World Trade Center* (Hollywood, CA: Paramount Pictures, 2006).

77. Dylan Avery (writer), *Loose Change 9/11: An American Coup* (location details unavailable: Louder Than Words, 2005).

78. Michael Moore (writer), *Fahrenheit 9/11* (location details unavailable: Fellowship Adventure Group, 2004).

79. John Law, *After Method*, 88.

80. Emphasis in original. Ibid.

81. Ibid, 90.

82. My emphasis. Ibid.

83. Ibid, 92.

84. Gabourey Sidibe, available at http://digg.com/celebrity/Precious_Star_Gabourey_Sidibe_The_Money_Shot_Dsheray_Dis?utm_source=feedburner&utm_medium=feed&utm_campaign=Feed%3A+digg%2Ftopic%2Fcelebrity%2Fupcoming+(Upcoming+in+Celebrity), retrieved on 9 March 2010.

85. In pornography, the money shot is the shot that captures a man ejaculating. More generally, in film it refers to the moment that the audience paid to see.

86. George W. Bush in BBC News, "US Marks Seventh 9/11 Anniversary", *BBC News*, 11 September 2008, available at http://news.bbc.co.uk/2/hi/americas/7609636.stm, retrieved on 19 August 2009.

87. Ibid.

88. Ibid.

Chapter 2

1. My emphasis. Joseph Conrad's preface to *The Secret Agent* (London, Vintage Books, [1920] 2007), xxi.

2. Andy Wachowski and Lana Wachowski (directors), *The Matrix* (Hollywood, CA: Silver Pictures, 1999).

3. Ibid.

4. Jean Baudrillard, *Simulacra and Simulation* (Ann Arbor: The University of Michigan Press, 1994).

5. Ibid, 1.

6. Emphasis in original. Ibid.

7. Slavoj Žižek, *Welcome to the Desert of the Real!: Five Essays on September 11 and Related Dates* (London: Verso, 2002).

8. Alain Badiou in Slavoj Žižek, *Welcome to the Desert of the Real!*, 5.

9. Emphasis in original. Slavoj Žižek, *Welcome to the Desert of the Real!*, 11.

10. Brian Jenkins, 'The Future Course of International Terrorism', in Paul Wilkinson and Alasdair Stewart (eds), *Contemporary Research on Terrorism* (Aberdeen: Aberdeen University Press, 1987).

11. Rod Plotnik, *Introduction to Psychology*, 7th Edn (Southbank, VIC: Thomson Wadsworth, 2005), 232.

12. Slavoj Žižek, *Welcome to the Desert of the Real!*, 11.

13. Jean Baudrillard, *The Spirit of Terrorism and Requiem for the Twin Towers* (London: Verso, 2002).

14. Toby Miller, "Being Ignorant, Living in Manhattan", 2002, available at www.portalcomunicacion.com/bcn2002/n_eng/contents/11/miller.pdf, retrieved on 1 February 2007; Michael Barnett, "From Me to We… and Back Again: Returning to Business as Usual", *Journal of Management Inquiry*, 2002, 11(3), 249-252.

15. Jean Baudrillard, *The Spirit of Terrorism*, 28-29.

16. Ibid, 3-4.

17. Slavoj Žižek, *Welcome to the Desert of the Real!*, 11.

18. Ibid.

19. Ibid.

20. Maria Tumarkin, *Traumascapes: The Power and Fate of Places Transformed by Tragedy* (Carlton, VIC: Melbourne University Press, 2005).

21. Ibid, 11.

22. Ibid, 12.

23. Ibid.

24. Zygmunt Bauman, *Liquid Life* (Cambridge: Polity, 2005).

25. Georg Simmel, "The Metropolis and Mental Life", in *On Individuality and Social Forms: Selected Writings* (Chicago: The University of Chicago Press, [1903] 1971), 324.

26. Ibid, 325.

27. Zillah Eisenstein, *Sexual Decoys: Gender, Race and War in Imperial Democracy* (London: Zed Books, 2007), xvii.

28. See Perri Campbell and Peter Kelly, "'Explosions and Examinations': Growing Up Female in Post-Saddam Iraq", *Journal of Youth Studies*, 2009, 12(1), 21-38.

29. Erich Fromm, *The Sane Society* (London: Routledge, [1956] 2008), 139-140.

30. Jennifer Edkins, "Forget Trauma? Response to September 11", *International Relations*, 2002, 16(2), 243.

31. Ibid.

32. See http://www.rialto.com.au/jd/jadehttp.dll?EbdMulti_www_01, retrieved on 25 February 2010.

33. See http://www.southerncrossstation.net.au/, retrieved on 25 February 2010.

34. See http://www.etihadstadium.com.au/, retrieved on 25 February 2010.

35. Luke Howie, *Terrorism, the Worker and the City: Simulations and Security in a Time of Terror* (Surrey: Gower/Ashgate, 2009); Luke Howie, *Terrorsex: Witnesses and the Reanimation of 9/11 as Image-event, Commodity and Pornography*, unpublished PhD thesis, Monash University, January 2008.

36. Luke Howie, *Terrorism, the Worker and the City.*

37. Patrick in Luke Howie, *Terrorism, the Worker and the City*, 117.

38. Paul in Luke Howie, *Terrorism, the Worker and the City*, 121, 129.

39. My emphasis. Price, interviewed on February 21, 2005. Defense employee.

40. My emphasis. Patrick in Luke Howie, *Terrorism, the Worker and the City*, 117.

41. Patrick in Luke Howie, *Terrorism, the Worker and the City*, 117.

42. Australian Human Right Commission, "Fact Sheet: Australian Muslims", available at http://www.hreoc.gov.au/racial_discrimination/isma/consultations/facts/fact_muslim.html, retrieved on 3 May 2010.

43. Paul in Luke Howie, *Terrorism, the Worker and the City*, 118.

44. Timothy, interviewed on 15 March 2005. Legal employee.

45. My emphasis. Paul in Luke Howie, *Terrorism, the Worker and the City*, 120.

46. Ibid.

47. Timothy in Luke Howie, *Terrorism, the Worker and the City*, 127.

48. Marcus in Luke Howie, *Terrorism, the Worker and the City*, 127.

49. Allen in *Terrorism, the Worker and the City*, 141.

50. Darrell West and Marion Orr, "Managing Citizen Fears: Public Attitudes Toward Urban Terrorism", *Urban Affairs Review*, 2005, 41(1), 93.

51. H.V. Savitch, "Does 9-11 Portend a New Paradigm for Cities?", *Urban Affairs Review*, 2003, 39(1), 107.

52. "Speculator" by *Insurge* from the album *Power to the Poison People* (Crows Nest, NSW: Warner Music Australia, 1996).

53. "51%" by *Insurge* from the album *Power to the Poison People* (Crows Nest, NSW: Warner Music Australia, 1996).

54. David Whittaker, *Terrorism: Understanding the Global Threat* (Harlow, UK: Pearson Longman, 2007).

55. Ibid, 27.

56. Luke Howie, *Terrorism, the Worker and the City*.

57. Slavoj Žižek, *First As Tragedy, Then As Farce* (London: Verso, 2009).

58. Ward Churchill, ""Some People Push Back": On the Justice of Roosting Chickens", available at http://www.kersplebedeb.com/mystuff/s11/churchill.html, 2003, retrieved on 3 July 2008.

59. Bryan Turner, *Vulnerability and Human Rights* (Pennsylvania: The Pennsylvania State University Press, 2006), 26.

Chapter 3

1. Denise Kiernan and Joseph D'Agnese, *The Official CTU Operations Manual* (Philadelphia: Quirk Books, 2007), 57. This is a fictional manual and an artifact from the popular counterterrorism themed television show, *24*, that tells the story of Special Agent Jack Bauer from the Los Angeles Domestic Unit of the CTU (Counterterrorism Unit).

2. "Remember, remember", available at http://www.rhymes.org.uk/remember_remember_the_5th_november.htm, retrieved on 20 April 2009.

3. Somini Sengupta, "At Least 100 Dead in India Terror Attacks", *The New York Times*, 26 November 2008, available at http://www.nytimes.com/2008/11/27/world/asia/27mumbai.html, retrieved on 15 March 2010.

4. Paul Cornish, "The Age of "Celebrity Terrorism", *BBC News*, 30 November 2008, available at http://news.bbc.co.uk/go/pr/fr/-/2/hi/south_asia/7755684.stm, retrieved on 23 July 2009.

5. My emphasis. Ibid.

6. Ibid; Alexandra Colen, "Paris Hilton Terrorism", *The Brussels Journal*, 2008, available http://www.brusselsjournal.com/node/3673, retrieved on 29 May 2009.

7. BBC News, "Toll Climbs in Egyptian Attacks", *BBC News*, 23 July 2005, available at http://news.bbc.co.uk/2/hi/middle_east/4709491.stm, retrieved on 15 March 2010.

8. Clive Williams, *Terrorism Explained: The Facts About Terrorism and Terrorist Groups* (Sydney: New Holland, 2004), 14.

9. Andy Wachowski and Lana Wachowski (screenplay writers), *V For Vendetta* (Burbank: Warner Bros. Pictures, 2005).

10. Walter Laqueur, *The Age of Terrorism* (Boston: Little, Brown and Company, 1987), 174

11. Perri Campbell and Peter Kelly, ""Explosions and Examinations": Growing Up Female in Post-Saddam Iraq", *Journal of Youth Studies*, 2009, 12, 22.

12. Denise Kiernan and Joseph D'Agnese, *The Official CTU Operations Manual*, 58.

13. Graeme Turner, *Understanding Celebrity* (Los Angeles: Sage, 2004); Toby Miller, *Sportsex* (Philadelphia: Temple University Press, 2002); Toby Miller, *Makeover Nation: The United States of Reinvention* (Columbus: The Ohio State University Press, 2008); Ellis Cashmore, *Celebrity/Culture* (Abingdon: Routledge, 2006).

14. Graeme Turner, *Understanding Celebrity*; Graeme Turner, "Tabloidisation, Journalism and the Possibility of Critique", *International Journal of Cultural Studies*, 1999, 2, 59-76; Graeme Turner, "The Mass Production of Celebrity: "Celetoids", Reality TV and the "Demotic Turn"", *International Journal of Cultural Studies*, 2006, 9, 153-165.

15. Graeme Turner, "The Mass Production of Celebrity", 153; Graeme Turner, *Understanding Celebrity*.

16. Graeme Turner, "The Mass Production of Celebrity", 153.

17. Ibid, 154.

18. Paul Cornish, "The Age of "Celebrity Terrorism"".

19. Luke Howie, *Terrorism, the Worker and the City: Simulations and Security in a Time of Terror* (Surrey: Gower/Ashgate, 2009), 5.

20. Paul Cornish, "The Age of "Celebrity Terrorism"".

21. Brian Jenkins, "The Future Course of International Terrorism", in Paul Wilkinson and A. Stewart (eds), *Contemporary Research on Terrorism* (Aberdeen: Aberdeen University Press, 1987), 583.

22. John Horgan, *The Psychology of Terrorism*, (London: Routledge, 2005), 3; Nehemia Friedland and Ariel Merari, "The Psychological Impact of Terrorism: A Double-Edged Sword", *Political Psychology*, 1985, 6, 592.

23. Alexandra Colen, "Paris Hilton Terrorism".

24. Ibid.

25. Ben Perrin, "Gauntlet Opinions – Celebrity Terrorism", *The Gauntlet*, 11 September 1998, available at http://thegauntlet.ca/a/story/4184, retrieved on 15 March 2010.

26. Ibid.

27. Ibid.

28. Brigitte Nacos, *Mass-Mediated Terrorism: The Central Role of the Media in Terrorism and Counterterrorism* (Lanham: Rowman and Littlefield Publishers, 2002), 89.

29. Ibid; Brigitte Nacos, *Terrorism & the Media: From the Iran Hostage Crisis to the Oklahoma City Bombing* (New York: Columbia University Press, 1994).

30. Brigitte Nacos, *Mass-Mediated Terrorism*, 88-94.

31. Ibid, 93.

32. Ibid.

33. Luke Howie, "Australia's History of Terrorism: Institutionalized Discrimination and the Response of the Mob", in Sean Brawley (ed), *Doomed To Repeat? Terrorism and the Lessons of History* (Washington D.C.: New Academia), 251-276.

34. James Button, "They Swear to Save Lives", *The Age*, 4 July 2007, 1.

35. Carly Crawford and Fiona Hudson, "Aussie Swoop as Police Believe They Have Cracked a Ring of ... TERROR DOCTORS", *Herald Sun*, 4 July 2007, 1.

36. Greg Pemberton, "Bombs Aimed at Heart of Democracy", *The Australian*, 4 July 2007, 14.

37. For a more detailed account see my chapter "Australia's History of Terrorism: Institutionalized Discrimination and the Response of the Mob" in Sean Brawley's (ed) *Doomed To Repeat? Terrorism and the Lessons of History* (Washington D.C.: New Academia), 251-276.

38. Carter Bays in Dylan Callaghan, "Those Were the Days", *Writers Guild of America*, available from http://www.wga.org/content/default.aspx?id=3118, 2009, retrieved on 22 April 2009.

39. BBC News, "Gunmen Shoot Sri Lanka Cricketers", *BBC News*, 3 March 2009, available at http://news.bbc.co.uk/go/pr/fr/-/2/hi/south_asia/7920260.stm, retrieved on 8 May 2009.

40. Brad West, "Collective Memory and Crisis: The 2002 Bali Bombings, National Heroic Archetypes and the Counter-narrative of Cosmopolitan Nationalism", *Journal of Sociology*, 2008, 44, 337-353.

41. Hollie McKay, "Is Singer Heather Schmid Being Targeted by Terrorists?", *Fox News*, 18 March 2009, available at http://www.foxnews.com/story/0,2933,509649,00.html, retrieved on 27 July 2009.

42. Heather Schmid in Ibid.

43. *Haaretz*, "Muslim Leader Threatens to Kill Paul McCartney Over Israel Gig", *Haaretz.com*, available at http://www.haaretz.com/hasen/spages/1020917.html, 2008, retrieved on 8 June 2009.

44. David Miller and Tom Mills, "The Terror Experts and the Mainstream Media: The Expert Nexus and its Dominance in the News Media", *Critical Studies on Terrorism*, 2009, 2(3), 414.

45. Ibid, 415.

46. I feel the need to clarify these comments. I do not intend to suggest that the scholars who rank highly on Miller and Mills study are, by definition, pandering to media demands. Indeed, many of the scholars on this list I consider to be of the highest quality and some are my friends. A Google Scholar search for Clive Williams, for example, will produce fewer returns than the same search conducted for Francis Fukuyama. But Clive Williams is a terror expert of the highest calibre with extensive field and intelligence experience combined with a complete knowledge of the terror studies academic canon. Others have accomplished little in the field and are certainly guilty of pandering to media requests.

47. Kevin Toolis, "Rise of the Terrorist Professors", *New Statesman*, 14 June 2004, available at http://www.newstatesman.com/print/200406140015, retrieved on 5 March 2010.

48. Ibid.

49. Petra Bartosiewicz, "Experts in Terror", *The Nation*, 17 January 2008, available at http://www.thenation.com/doc/20080204/bartosiewicz/print, retrieved on 5 March 2010.

50. "Dick Destiny", "Celebrity Terrorism Expert", *Dick Destiny*, August 28, 2009, available at http://www.dickdestiny.com/blog/2009/08/celebrity-terrorism-expert-always-there.html, retrieved on 5 March 2010.

51. Ibid.

52. Ibid.

53. Denise Kiernan and Joseph D'Agnese, *The Official CTU Operations Manual*, 157.

54. See for an account of what is at stake Aaron Barlow, *The Rise of the Blogosphere* (Westport, Conn: Praeger, 2007); Brian McNair, *Cultural Chaos: Journalism, News, and Power in a Globalised World* (New York: Routledge, 2006); Perri Campbell and Peter Kelly, "Explosions and Examinations".

55. See Brigitte Nacos, *Mass-Mediated Terrorism*; Brigitte Nacos, *Terrorism & the Media*; Philip Seib, *The Al Jazeera Effect: How the New Global Media are Reshaping World Politics* (Washington D.C.: Potomac, 2008); Jeffory Clymer, *America's Culture of Terrorism: Violence, Capitalism and the Written Word* (Chapel Hill: University of North Carolina Press, 2003); Anthony Kubiak, *Stages of Terror: Terrorism, Ideology, and Coercion as Theatre History* (Bloomington: Indiana University Press, 1991); Luke Howie, *Terrorism, the*

Worker and the City; Gabriel Weimann and Conrad Winn, *The Theatre of Terror: Mass Media and International Terrorism* (New York: Longman, 1994).

56. Piers Morgan in Graeme Turner, *Understanding Celebrity*, 128.

57. "Irco", "The Age of "Celebrity Terrorism"", 1 December 2008, available at http://digg.com/world_news/The_age_of_celebrity_terrorism, retrieved on 23 July 2009.

58. Graeme Turner, *Understanding Celebrity*, 128.

59. Paul Cornish, "The Age of "Celebrity Terrorism"".

60. Ibid.

61. "domiciliphile", "The Age of "Celebrity Terrorism"", 30 November 2008, available at http://digg.com/world_news/The_age_of_celebrity_terrorism, retrieved on 23 July 2009.

62. See http://www.presscouncil.org.au/snpma/snpma2007/ch02_2_snpma2007.html, retrieved on 8 April 2010.

63. Herald Sun, "Four Arrests in Terror Swoop", *Herald Sun*, 4 August 2009.

64. Ibid.

65. Ibid.

66. Thomas Hunter, "Counter-terrorism Raids Across Melbourne", *Brisbane Times*, 4 August 2009, available at http://www.brisbanetimes.com.au/national/counterterrorism-raids-across-melbourne-20090804-e7iu.html, retrieved on 17 March 2010; Peter Gregory and Thomas Hunter, "Counter-terrorism Raids Across Melbourne", *The Age*, 4 August 2009, retrieved on http://www.theage.com.au/national/counterterrorism-raids-across-melbourne-20090804-e7i5.html, retrieved on 17 March 2010.

67. Herald Sun, "Four Arrests in Terror Swoop".

68. Ibid.

69. Phillip Coorey, "Increased Terror Risk From Within", *The Sydney Morning Herald*, 23 February 2010, 1.

70. Denise Kiernan and Joseph D'Agnese, *The Official CTU Operations Manual*, 155.

71. Edward Neumeier (writer of screenplay) and Robert A. Heinlein (writer of book), *Starship Troopers* (Culver City, CA: TriStar Pictures, 1997).

72. Judd Aptow in "Chauncey Billups" [I understand this to be a pseudonym, and not literally the NBA basketballer for the Denver Nuggets], "Celebrity Obsession and Terrorism", available at http://blogcritics.org/scitech/article/celebrity-obsession-and-terrorism/, 2005, retrieved on 5 March 2010.

73. Ibid.

74. See Jean Baudrillard, *The Spirit of Terrorism and Requiem for the Twin Towers* (London: Verso, 2002), 3-4.

Chapter 4

1. Jenny Edkins, "Forget Trauma? Response to September 11", *International Relations*, 2002, 16(2), 243.

2. David Crane and Marta Kauffman (creators), *Friends* [television series 1994-2004] (Burbank: Warner Brothers, 1994).

3. David Zurawik, "Era of Smiles Fading Away", *Baltimore Sun*, 2 May 2004, available at www.baltimoresun.com/entertainment/tv/bal-as.friends02may02,0,1061507.story, retrieved on 7 July 2008.

4. Slavoj Žižek, *Violence: Six Sideways Reflections* (New York: Picador, 2008), 45-46.

5. Slavoj Žižek, *Welcome to the Desert of the Real! Five Essays on September 11 and Related Dates* (London: Verso, 2002); Slavoj Žižek, *The Pervert's Guide to Cinema: Parts 1, 2, 3* (London: A Lone Star, Mischief Films, Amoeba Film Production, 2006).

6. Slavoj Žižek, *Welcome to the Desert of the Real!*, 10.

7. Paolo Fusar-Poli, Oliver Howes, Lucia Valmaggia and Philip McGuire, "'Truman' Signs and Vulnerability to Psychosis", *The British Journal of Psychiatry*, 2008, 193, 168; Peter Weir (director), *The Truman Show* (Hollywood, CA: Paramount Pictures, 1998).

8. My emphasis. Slavoj Žižek, *Welcome to the Desert of the Real!*, 13.

9. Ibid.

10. Ibid.

11. Ibid.

12. Jeffrey Prager, "Healing from History: Psychoanalytic Considerations on Traumatic Pasts and Social Repair", 2008, *European Journal of Social Theory*, 11(3), 408.

13. Zygmunt Bauman, *Liquid Fear* (Cambridge: Polity, 2006), 17.

14. Ibid.

15. Ibid.

16. See also Slavoj Žižek, *Enjoy Your Symptom! Jacques Lacan in Hollywood and Out*, 2nd edn (New York: Routledge, 2001); Slavoj Žižek (ed), *Everything You Always Wanted to Know About Lacan (But Were Afraid to Ask Hitchcock)* (London: Verso, 2002); Slavoj Žižek, "The Matrix: Or, Two Sides of Perversion", in William Irwin (ed), *The Matrix and Philosophy: Welcome to the Desert of the Real* (Chicago: Open Court, 2002), 240-266; Slavoj Žižek, *The Pervert's Guide to Cinema*; Slavoj Žižek, *Violence*.

17. Emphasis in original. Erich Fromm, *The Sane Society* (London: Routledge, [1956] 2008), 141.

18. My emphasis. Ibid, 141-142.

19. Ibid.

20. Jean Baudrillard, *The Spirit of Terrorism and Requiem for the Twin Towers* (London: Verso, 2002), 4.

21. Rob Hirst, *Willie's Bar & Grill: A Rock 'n' Roll Tour of North America in the Age of Terror* (Sydney: Picador, 2003), 10.

22. Ibid, 10-11.

23. Lukas Szymanek, ""Friends" Not Forever in Television", *Lumino Magazine*, 15 April 2004, available at http://www.luminomagazine.com/mw/content/view/921/4, retrieved on 7 July 2008.

24. Piotr Sztrompka, "Cultural Trauma: The Other Face of Social Change", *European Journal of Social Theory*, 2000, 3(4), 449-466; Howard Waitzkin and H. Magaña, "The Black Box in Somatization: Unexplained Physical Symptoms, Culture, and Narratives of Trauma", *Social Science and Medicine*, 1997, 45(6), 811-825; Jeffrey C. Alexander, Ron Eyerman, Bernhard Giesen, Neil J. Smelser, Piotr Sztrompka, *Cultural Trauma* (Berkeley: University of California Press, 2000); Jeffrey C. Alexander, Ron Eyerman and Bernhard Giesen, *Cultural Trauma and Collective Identity* (Berkeley: University of California Press, 2004); Judith Herman, *Trauma and Recovery* (New York: Basic Books, 1992); Cathy Caruth (ed), *Trauma: Explorations in Memory* (Baltimore: Johns Hopkins University Press, 1995); Cathy Caruth, *Unclaimed Experience: Trauma, Narrative, and History* (Baltimore: Johns Hopkins University Press, 1996); Arthur G. Neal, *National Trauma and Collective Memory* (Armonk: M.E. Sharpe, 1998); Michael S. Roth, *Memory, Trauma and the Construction of History* (New York: Columbia University Press, 1995); Maria Tumarkin, *Traumascapes: The Power and Fate of Places Transformed by Tragedy* (Carlton: Melbourne University Press, 2005); Slavoj Žižek, *On Belief* (London: Routledge, 2001); Slavoj Žižek, *The Parallax View* (Cambridge: The MIT Press, 2006); Slavoj Žižek (ed), *Everything You Always Wanted to Know About Lacan*, and, to some extent, Roland Barthes, *Image – Music – Text* (New York: Hill and Wang, 1978), 28-31 for his account of the traumatic image.

25. Roland Barthes, *Image – Music – Text*, 28-31.

26. Slavoj Žižek, *Welcome to the Desert of the Real!*; Slavoj Žižek, *Violence*; Jean Baudrillard, *The Spirit of Terrorism*.

27. Slavoj Žižek, *Violence*, 45-46.

28. My emphasis. Ibid.

29. I argue that this same fetishistic disavowal is apparent in post-9/11 M. Night Shyamalan movies. Notably, Žižek explores the meaning of Shyamalan's *The Village* in a similar context. This film is centered on life in a paranoid and gated community. I suggest that this paranoia can be similarly viewed in post-9/11 episodes of *Friends*.

30. See Luke Howie, *Terrorism, the Worker and the City: Simulations and Security in a Time of Terror* (Surrey: Gower/Ashgate, 2009), 5.

31. Slavoj Žižek, *On Belief* , 32.

32. Ibid, 47.

33. Maria Tumarkin, *Traumascapes*, 23-53.

34. Toby Miller, "Being Ignorant, Living in Manhattan", 2002, available at www.portalcomunicacion.com/bcn2002/n_eng/contents/11/miller.pdf, retrieved on 1 February 2007; Toby Miller, *Cultural Citizenship: Cosmopolitanism, Consumerism, and Television in a Neoliberal Age* (Philadelphia: Temple University Press, 2007).

35. Toby Miller, "Being Ignorant".

36. Ward Churchill, ""Some People Push Back": On the Justice of Roosting Chickens", 2003, available at http://www.kersplebedeb.com/mystuff/s11/churchill.html, retrieved on 3 July 2008; Ward Churchill, *On the Justice of Roosting Chickens: Reflections on the Consequences of U.S. Imperial Arrogance and Criminality* (Oakland, CA: AK Press, 2003).

37. Ward Churchill, ""Some People Push Back"".

38. Zygmunt Bauman, *Liquid Fear*, 97. Bauman quotes here from Arundhati Roy, "L'Empire n'est pas invulnérable", *Manière de Voir*, 2004, 75(June-July), 63-66.

39. Darren Star (creator), *Sex and the City* [television series 1998-2004] (New York: HBO, 1998).

40. Lewis Whittington, "Sex and the City – The Final Season", *Culturevulture.net: Choices for the Cognoscenti*, no date, available at http://www.culturevulture.net/Television/SexandtheCity.htm, retrieved on 8 July 2008.

41. David Zurawik, "Era of Smiles Fading Away".

42. Jean Baudrillard, *Simulacra and Simulation* (Ann Arbor: University of Michigan Press, 1994).

43. Carol D. Lee, Erica Rosenfeld, Ruby Mendenhall, Ama Rivers and Brendesha Tynes, "Cultural Modeling as a Frame for Narrative Analysis", in Colette Daiute and Cynthia Lightfoot (eds), *Narrative Analysis: Studying the Development of Individuals in Society* (Thousand Oaks: Sage, 2004), 39.

44. Catherine Kohler Riessman, *Narrative Analysis* (Newbury Park: Sage, 1993), 1.

45. Mark Freeman, "Data are Everywhere: Narrative Criticism in the Literature of Experience", in Colette Daiute and Cynthia Lightfoot (eds), *Narrative Analysis: Studying the Development of Individuals in Society* (Thousand Oaks: Sage, 2004), 63.

46. My emphasis. Elizabeth Grosz, *Architecture From the Outside: Essays on Virtual and Real Space* (Cambridge: The MIT Press, 2001), 57.

47. Ibid, 57-58.

48. Elizabeth Grosz, *Space, Time and Perversion: The Politics of Bodies* (St Leonards: Allen & Unwin, 1995), 105.

49. David Crane and Marta Kauffman (creators), "The One After "I Do"", *Friends*, season eight, episode one (Burbank: Warner Brothers Studios, 2001).

50. David Crane and Marta Kauffman (creators), "The One Where Rachel Tells", *Friends*, season eight, episode three (Burbank: Warner Brothers Studios, 2001).

51. TV.com, "The One Where Rachel Tells...", *TV.com*, 2008, available at http://www.tv.com/friends/the-one-where-rachel-tells.../episode/73775/summary.html, retrieved on 4 May 2008.

52. Rob Hirst, *Willie's Bar & Grill*, 10.

53. Ibid.

54. See Erich Fromm, *The Sane Society*, 47-48; and see Robert Greenwald, *Outfoxed: Rupert Murdoch's War on Journalism* (Columbia, SC: Carolina Productions, 2004); Danny Schechter, *WMD: Weapons of Mass Deception* (Canoga Park, CA: Cinema Libre, 2004).

55. Barack Obama in Associated Press, "Barack Obama Stops Wearing American Flag Lapel Pin", *Fox News*, 4 October 2007, available at http://www.foxnews.com/printer_friendly_story/0,3566,299439,00.html, retrieved on 11 November 2008.

56. Associated Press, "Barack Obama Stops Wearing American Flag Lapel Pin".

57. David Crane and Marta Kauffman (creators), "The One Where Joey Dates Rachel", season eight, episode twelve (Burbank: Warner Brothers Studios, 2001).

58. Michael Burke in Tim Sumner, "Capt. Burke Died on 9/11 at the Hands of "Enemy Combatants"", *9/11 Families for a Safe & Strong America*, 2007, available at http://www.911familiesforamerica.org/?p=341, retrieved on 10 July 2008; CNN, "September 11 – A Memorial", *CNN.com*, 2002, available at http://www.cnn.com/SPECIALS/2001/memorial/people/2144.html, retrieved on 10 July 2008.

59. My emphasis. David Zurawik, "Era of Smiles Fading Away".

60. Slavoj Žižek, *Violence*, 45-46.

61. My emphasis. Slavoj Žižek, *Welcome to the Desert of the Real!*, 13.

62. Rembrandts, "I'll Be There For You", theme music to *Friends*, lyrics available at http://www.lyricsondemand.com/onehitwonders/illbethere-foryoulyrics.html, retrieved on 8 July 2008.

Chapter 5

1. Søren Kierkegaard, *Fear and Trembling/Repetition: Kierkegaard's Writings, VI*, trans. by H. V. Hong and E. H. Hong (Princeton, NJ: Princeton University Press, 1983), 158.

2. *The Book of Pythia* in David Kyle Johnson, ""A Story that is Told Again and Again, and Again": Recurrence, Providence and Freedom", in Jason T. Eberl (ed.) *Battlestar Galactica and Philosophy: Knowledge Here Begins Out There* (Malden, MA: Blackwell, 2008), 181.

3. Bill Gorman, "*Battlestar Galactica* Finale Blasts Away the Competition", 2009, available at http://tvbythenumbers.com/2009/03/24/battlestar-galactica-finale-blasts-away-the-competition/15054, retrieved on 18 January 2010.

4. Slavoj Žižek, *Violence: Six Sideways Reflections* (London: Profile Books, 2008), 1-13.

5. Ibid, 1.

6. Ibid.

7. Interestingly, Žižek further distinguishes symbolic violence along the lines of the subjective/objective distinction. There are language acts that are direct violent outburst such as discrimination and verbal abuse, but there are also structural features of language that impose more subtle, objective language violence. A word like "terrorism" is a particularly tendentious example of this. The word "terrorism" has a meaning buried deep behind its negative connotations and its elitist assumptions (ie: the US State Department describes those who oppose the USA as "terrorists", but when the US military drops bombs on Baghdad in an operation called "Shock and Awe" it is, somehow, not "officially" terrorism).

8. Slavoj Žižek, *Violence*, 1.

9. Slavoj Žižek, *The Metastases of Enjoyment: Six Essays on Women and Causality* (London: Verso, [1994] 2005), 16-17.

10. Ibid, 16.

11. Slavoj Žižek, *The Metastases of Enjoyment*, 18; Slavoj Žižek, "You May!", *London Review of Books*, 1999, 21(6), 3-6, available at http://www.lrb.co.uk/v21/n06/slavoj-zizek/you-may, retrieved 11 December 2007.

12. Emphasis in original. Slavoj Žižek, *The Parallax View* (Cambridge: The MIT Press, 2006), 368-369.

13. Ibid, 367.

14. Despite the perpetrators of suicide terrorism dying in the act of carrying them out, the shock of this type of subjective violence somehow provides a license to blame someone else.

15. Noam Chomsky, *The Culture of Terrorism* (Boston: South End Press, 1988), 5-7, 11-24.

16. Michael Dudley, "*Battlestar Galactica*: Immersion Therapy for Post 9/11 World", available at http://www.alternet.org/module/printversion/133419, 2009, retrieved on 14 January 2010.

17. Susan Faludi, *The Terror Dream: Fear and Fantasy in Post-9/11 America* (Melbourne: Scribe, 2008); Toby Miller, *Cultural Citizenship: Cosmopolitanism, Consumerism, and Television in A Neoliberal Age* (Philadelphia: Temple University Press, 2007); John Mueller, *Overblown: How Politicians and the Terrorism Industry Inflate National Security Threats, and Why We Believe Them* (New York: Free Press, 2006); Sut Jhally and Jeremy Earp (eds.), *Hijacking*

Catastrophe: 9/11, Fear and the Selling of American Empire (Northampton: Olive Branch Press, 2004).

18. Brian L. Ott, "(Re)Framing Fear: Equipment for Living in a Post-9/11 World", in Tiffany Potter and C.W. Marshall (eds.), *Cylons in America: Critical Studies in* Battlestar Galactica (New York: Continuum, 2008), 13.

19. Brian Jenkins, "The Future Course of International Terrorism", in Paul Wilkinson and Alasdair M. Stewart (eds.), *Contemporary Research on Terrorism* (Aberdeen: Aberdeen University Press, 1987), 581-589.

20. Brian L. Ott, "(Re)Framing Fear", 14; Ned Martel, "Television Review; The Cylons are Back and Humanity is in Deep Trouble", *New York Times*, 8 December 2003, available at http://www.nytimes.com/2003/12/08/arts/television-review-the-cylons-are-back-and-humanity-is-in-deep-trouble.html, retrieved on 11 December 2009.

21. Brian L. Ott, "(Re)Framing Fear", 17.

22. Slavoj Žižek, *The Ticklish Subject: The Absent Centre of Political Ontology* (London: Verso, 1999), 322-323; Mark Andrejevic, "The Body, Torture, and the Decline of Symbolic Efficiency", *Politics and Culture*, no date, available at http://aspen.conncoll.edu/politicsandculture/page.cfm?key=538, retrieved on 20 January 2010; Luke Howie, "Representing Terrorism: Reanimating Post-9/11 New York City", *International Journal of Žižek Studies*, 2009, 3(3), available at http://zizekstudies.org/index.php/ijzs/issue/view/15, retrieved on 5 January 2010.

23. Brian L. Ott, "(Re)Framing Fear"; Erika Johnson-Lewis, "Torture, Terrorism, and Other Aspects of Human Nature", in Tiffany Potter and C.W. Marshall (eds.), *Cylons in America: Critical Studies in* Battlestar Galactica (New York: Continuum, 2008); Isabel Pinedo, "Playing With Fire Without Getting Burned: Blowback Re-imagined", in Josef Steiff and Tristan D. Tamplin (eds.), Battlestar Galactica *and Philosophy: Mission Accomplished Or Mission Frakked Up?* (Chicago: Open Court, 2008).

24. Slavoj Žižek, *Violence*, 151-152.

25. Slavoj Žižek, *Welcome to the Desert of the Real!: Five Essays on September 11 and Related Dates* (London: Verso, 2002), 12.

26. See http://www.imdb.com/title/tt1405819/, retrieved on 11 December 2009.

27. Louis Melançon, "Secrets and Lies: Balancing Security and Democracy in the Colonial Fleet", in Josef Steiff and Tristan D. Tamplin (eds.), Battlestar Galactica *and Philosophy: Mission Accomplished or Mission Frakked Up?* (Chicago: Open Court, 2008), 211.

28. Marita Grabiak and Ronald D. Moore, "Water", *Battlestar Galactica*, episode two, season one (Hollywood: Universal Studios, 2004).

29. In a final irony, Tyrol also turns out to be a Cylon sleeper agent. But, like Boomer, he identifies with his humanity and indeed, as the

viewer later learns, Tyrol is one of the "Final Five" – an original model of humanoid Cylons that had long desired lasting peace between Cylons and humans.

30. Michael Taylor (writer) and Michael Nankin (director), "The Ties That Bind", *Battlestar Galactica*, episode three, season four (Hollywood: Universal Studios, 2008).

31. Louis Melançon, "Secrets and Lies", 215.

32. Emphasis in original. Ibid, 215-216.

33. Jenny Freyd, "In the Wake of Terrorist Attack, Hatred May Mask Fear", *Analyses of Social Issues and Public Policy*, 2002, 2(1), 5-8.

34. Jenny Freyd, "In the Wake of Terrorist Attack", 5; L. Sixel, "EEOC Suit Claims Firing Prompted By Terrorism Fear", *Houston Chronicle.*, 2004, available at http://www.chron.com/cs/CDA/printstory.mpl/business/six-el/206095, retrieved 22 March 2004.

35. See also Daniel Pipes, "Sheik Obama and His Two Wars", available at http://www.danielpipes.org/, 2009, retrieved 3 January 2010.

36. Brian L. Ott, "(Re)Framing Fear", 17.

37. Erika Johnson-Lewis, "Torture, Terrorism, and Other Aspects of Human Nature", in Tiffany Potter and C.W. Marshall (eds.), *Cylons in America: Critical Studies in* Battlestar Galactica (New York: Continuum, 2008), 30.

38. Michael Taylor (writer) and Michael Nankin (director), "The Ties That Bind".

39. Tony Norman, "The Hilarious Dangerous World of Dave Chappelle", *Post-Gazette*, 2004, available at http://www.post-gazette.com/columnists/20040127normanp5.asp, retrieved on 22 January 2010.

40. Slavoj Žižek, *Violence*, 1; Slavoj Žižek, *The Parallax View*, 364-375.

41. A fact not fully accounted for until the release of the *Caprica* (2009) mini-series.

42. Eric Greene, "The Mirror Frakked: Reflections on *Battlestar Galactica*", in Richard Hatch (ed.), *So Say We All: An Unauthorized Collection of Thoughts and Opinions on* Battlestar Galactica (Dallas: Benbella Books, 2006), 8.

43. Georgio Agamben, *Homo Sacer: Sovereign Power and Bare Life*, trans. by D. Heller-Roazen (Stanford, CA: Stanford University Press, 1998).

44. Jim Casey, ""All This Has Happened Before": Repetition, Reimagination, and Eternal Return", in Tiffany Potter and C.W. Marshall (eds.), *Cylons in America: Critical Studies in* Battlestar Galactica (New York: Continuum, 2008); Erika Johnson-Lewis, "Torture, Terrorism, and Other Aspects of Human Nature"; Isabel Pinedo, "Playing With Fire".

45. Jim Casey, "All This Has Happened Before", 237.

46. Isabel Pinedo, "Playing With Fire".

47. Slavoj Žižek, *First as Tragedy, The as Farce* (London: Verso, 2009).

48..My emphasis. Ronald D. Moore and Christopher James (writers), *Battlestar Galactica* (Hollywood: Universal Studios, 2004).

49. Noam Chomsky, *September 11* (Crows Nest, NSW: Allen and Unwin, 2001).

50. Ibid, 18.

51. Bill O'Reilly in Robert Greenwald, *Outfoxed: Rupert Murdoch's War on Journalism* (London: The Disinformation Company, 2004).

52. Robert Sheer, *The Pornography of Power: Why Defense Spending Must be Cut* (New York: Twelve, 2008), 12-13.

53. Sylvester Stallone and Sheldon Lettich (writers), *Rambo III* (Culver City, CA: Tri Star Pictures, 1988).

54. Slavoj Žižek, "Foreword: Trotsky's *Terrorism and Communism*, or, Despair and Utopia in the Turbulent Year of 1920", in Leon Trotsky *Terrorism and Communism: A Reply to Karl Kautsky* (London: Verso, 2007), xvi.

55. Slavoj Žižek, *First as Tragedy*, 4; Slavoj Žižek, *Violence*, 20-21.

56. Slavoj Žižek, *First as Tragedy*, 3.

57. Emily Vencat and Ginanne Brownell in Slavoj Žižek, *First as Tragedy*, 4.

58. My emphasis. Slavoj Žižek, *First as Tragedy*, 4.

59. Ward Churchill, *On the Justice of Roosting Chickens: Reflections on the Consequences of U.S. Imperial Arrogance and Criminality* (Oakland, CA: AK Press, 2003); Ward Churchill, ""Some People Push Back": On the Justice of Roosting Chickens", 2003, available at http://wwwkersplebedeb.com/mystuff/s11/churchill.html, retrieved on 3 July 2008.

60. Ward Churchill, "Some People Push Back".

61. Slavoj Žižek, *First as Tragedy*, 5.

62. Doug Liman and Paul Greengrass, *The Bourne Trilogy: The Bourne Identity, The Bourne Supremacy, The Bourne Ultimatum* (Hollywood: Universal Studios, 2002-2007).

63. Slavoj Žižek, *Violence*, 3.

64. Simon Jenkins, "Indiscriminate Slaughter From the Air is a Barbarism that must be Abolished", *The Guardian*, 16 January 2009, available at http://www.guardian.co.uk/commentisfree/2009/jan/16/gaza-aerial-bombing-david-miliband/print, retrieved on 7 January 2010.

65. David Kilcullen, *The Accidental Guerilla: Fighting Small Wars in the Midst of a Big One* (Melbourne: Scribe, 2009).

Chapter 6

1. Robert Pinsky, "Impossible to Tell", in *The Figured Wheel: New and Collected Poems, 1966-1996* (New York: Farrar, Straus and Giroux, 1996).

Poem available at http://www.ibiblio.org/ipa/poems/pinsky/impossible_ to_tell.php, retrieved on 11 January 2010.

2. Julia Kristeva, "Stabat Mater", *Poetics Today*, 6(1-2), 1985, 133-152; Anthony Elliott, *Concepts of the Self*, 2nd edn (Cambridge: Polity, 2007, 121-122).

3. John Law, *After Method: Mess In Social Science Research* (London: Routledge, 2004), 1.

4. Slavoj Žižek, *Welcome to the Desert of the Real: Five Essays on September 11 and Related Dates* (London: Verso, 2002), 1-12.

5. Maria Tumarkin, *Traumascapes: The Power and Fate of Places Transformed by Tragedy* (Carlton: Melbourne University Press, 2005).

6. Jason Gay, "Dave at Peace: The Rolling Stone Interview", *Rollingstone.com*, available at http://www.rollingstone.com/news/story/22791344/ dave_at_peace_the_rolling_stone_interview/print, retrieved on 7 September 2009.

7. See, for example, David Niven, S. Robert Lichter and Daniel Amundson, "The Political Content of Late Night Comedy", *The Harvard International Journal of Press/Politics*, 8(3), 2003, 118-133. This article is a useful account of Letterman's influence during the 2000 US Presidential Elections.

8. David Letterman, *Late Show*, 17 September 2001, available at http:// video.google.com.au/videosearch?q=Letterman+post-9%2F11&hl= en&emb=0&aq=f#, retrieved on 7 May 2009. I transcribed this video but I also consulted a transcription that can be found at http://www.geocities.com/davidletterman82/LateShowTranscriptSeptember17th.html, retrieved on 15 May 2009.

9. Scott Derrickson (director), David Scarpa (screenplay) and Edmund H. North (screenplay, 1951), *The Day The Earth Stood Still* (Los Angeles: Twentieth Century Fox, 2008).

10. Emphasis in original. Erich Fromm, *The Sane Society* (London: Routledge, [1956] 2008), 140.

11. Ibid.

12. In Slavoj Žižek, *The Universal Exception: Selected Writings, Volume Two* (London: Continuum, 2006), 275.

13. Toby Miller, "Being Ignorant, Living in Manhattan", 2002, available at www.portalcomunicacion.com/bcn2002/n_eng/contents/11/miller.pdf, retrieved on 1 February 2007; Toby Miller, *Cultural Citizenship: Cosmopolitanism, Consumerism, and Television in a Neoliberal Age* (Philadelphia: Temple University Press, 2007); Ward Churchill, ""Some People Push Back": On the Justice of Roosting Chickens", 2003, available at http://www.kersplebedeb.com/mystuff/s11/churchill.html, retrieved on 3 July 2008; Ward Churchill, *On the Justice of Roosting Chickens: Reflections on the Consequences of U.S. Imperial Arrogance and Criminality* (Oakland, CA: AK Press, 2003).

14. Slavoj Žižek, *The Universal Exception*, 275

15. Ibid.

16. With thanks to my colleague in the Global Terrorism Research Centre (GTReC) Virginie André for talking me through the possible meanings of this phrase.

17. Howard Zinn, *Terrorism and War* (Crows Nest, NSW: Allen & Unwin, 2002); Noam Chomsky, *September 11* (Crows Nest, NSW: Allen & Unwin, 2001); Toby Miller, *Cultural Citizenship*.

18. Dan Rather on David Letterman, *Late Show*.

19. My emphasis. Ibid.

20. Toby Miller, "Being Ignorant".

21. Ziauddin Sardar and Merryl Wyn Davies, *Why Do People Hate America?* (Duxford: Icon Books, 2002), v.

22. Ibid, 5-38; Ziauddin Sardar and Merryl Wyn Davies, *Will America Change?* (Thriplow: Icon Books, 2008), 1-29.

23. Ziauddin Sardar and Merryl Wyn Davies, *Will America Change?*, 123.

24. James Poniewozik, "'West Wing': Terrorism 101", *Time*, Thursday 4 October 2001, available at http://www.time.com/time/printout/0,8816,178042,00.html, retrieved on 17 September 2009.

25. Sam Seeborn in Aaron Sorkin (writer), "Isaac and Ishmael", *The West Wing*, season three, episode 0 (a pre-season three special episode that is said to fall outside of *The West Wing* cannon), clip available at http://www.youtube.com/watch?v=NDsY8qCxLHQ, retrieved on 4 September 2009.

26. James Poniewozik, "'West Wing': Terrorism 101".

27. Louise Richardson, *What Terrorists Want: Understanding the Terrorist Threat* (London: John Murray, 2006), 44.

28. See any number of generalist books about terrorism or the IRA. I recommend Tim Pat Coogan, *The I.R.A* (London: Harper Collins, 2000); Louise Richardson, *What Terrorists Want*; Walter Laqueur, *No End To War: Terrorism in the Twenty-First Century* (New York: Continuum, 2003); Walter Laqueur, *The New Terrorism: Fanaticism and the Arms of Mass Destruction* (London: Phoenix Press, 1999).

29. Noam Chomsky, *September 11*.

30. Jody Baumgartner and Jonathan S. Morris, "*The Daily Show* Effect: Candidate Evaluations, Efficacy, and American Youth", *American Politics Research*, 34(3), 342.

31. Ibid, 341-367.

32. Dana Larsen, "Tal Host Tokers", *Cannabis Culture: Marijuana Magazine*, 25 May 2009, available at http://www.cannabisculture.com/articles/4284.html, retrieved on 10 November 2009.

33. John Stewart, "The Daily Show – First Broadcast After 9/11", available at http://www.buzznet.com/www/search/videos/speech/3401696/daily-show-first-broadcast-after/, retrieved on 4 September 2009. My transcription.

34. D. Fromkin, "The Strategy of Terrorism", *Foreign Affairs*, 53(4): 684-685.

35. Ulrich Beck and Elizabeth Beck-Gernsheim, *Individualization: Institutionalized Individualism and Its Social and Political Consequences* (London: Sage, 2002), 6.

36. Ibid.

37. Luke Howie, *Terrorism, the Worker and the City: Simulations and Security in a Time of Terror* (Surrey: Gower/Ashgate, 2009), 32.

38. Slavoj Žižek, *Welcome to the Desert of the Real!*, 135.

39. Jean Baudrillard, *Simulacra and Simulation* (Ann Arbor: The University of Michigan Press, 1994).

40. Slavoj Žižek, *Welcome to the Desert of the Real!*, 141.

41. Ibid, 141-142.

42. Giselinde Kuipers, ""Where Was King Kong When We Needed Him?" Public Discourse, Digital Disaster Jokes, and the Functions of Laughter After 9/11", *The Journal of American Culture*, 2005, 28(1), 70.

43. TV.Com, "The One Where Rachel Tells ...", *TV.com*, 2008, available at http://www.tv.com/friends/the-one-where-rachel-tells.../episode/73775/summary.html, retrieved on 4 May 2008.

44. Bill Oakley, Josh Weinstein and Jim Reardon, "The City of New York vs. Homer Simpson", *The Simpsons* – audio commentary special feature of season nine, episode one (Moore Park, NSW: Twentieth Century Fox, 2007).

45. Ibid.

46. Ibid.

47. Ibid.

48. Sarah Kay, *Žižek: A Critical Introduction* (Cambridge: Polity, 2003), 172.

49. Martin Heidegger, "The Thing", *Poetry, Language, Thought* (New York: Perennial Classics, 1971), 163-180.

50. Ibid, 165.

51. Ibid, 163.

52. Jean Baudrillard, *The Spirit of Terrorism and Requiem for the Twin Towers* (London: Verso, 2002), 5.

53. My emphasis. Ibid, 5.

54. Slavoj Žižek, *Welcome to the Desert of the Real!*, 12.

55. Jean Baudrillard, *The Spirit of Terrorism*, 5.

56. My emphasis. Ibid, 5.

57. Ward Churchill, "On the Justice of Roosting Chickens".

58. Walter Laqueur, *The New Terrorism*, 144.

59. See Slavoj Žižek, *Organs Without Bodies: On Deleuze and Consequences* (New York: Routledge, 2004), 87-93.

60. Bill Oakley, Josh Weinstein and Jim Reardon, "The City of New York vs. Homer Simpson".

61. Ibid.

62. Ibid.

63. Chris Turner, *Planet Simpson* (London: Ebury, 2005).

64. Nancy Kruse (director) and Marc Wilmore (writer), "Midnight RX", *The Simpsons*, episode 1606, available at http://www.wtso.net/movie/208-The_Simpsons_1606_Midnight_Rx.html, retrieved on 18 September 2009.

65. Steven Dean Moore (director) and Marc Wilmore (writer), "Mypods and Boomsticks", *The Simpsons*, episode 2007, available at http://www.wtso.net/movie/440-2007_Mypods_and_Boomsticks.html, retrieved on 17 September 2009.

66. Hussam Ayloush, Executive Director of the *Council on American-Islamic Relations*, letter to Matt Groening, the creator and director of *The Simpsons*, 3 December 2008, available at http://cair-california.org/images/stories/thank_you_letter_-_matt_groening.pdf, retrieved on 17 September 2009.

67. Steven Dean Moore (director) and Marc Wilmore (writer), "Mypods and Boomsticks".

68. Hussam Ayloush, letter to Matt Groening.

69. IMDb, "Simpsons Creator Defends Muslim Plot", available at http://www.imdb.com/news/ni0645713/, retrieved on 18 September 2009.

70. In Jeffrey Melnick, *9/11 Culture* (West Sussex: Wiley-Blackwell, 2009), 52.

71. Ibid.

72. Bryan Turner, *Vulnerability and Human Rights* (Pennsylvania: Pennsylvania University Press, 2006), 62.

73. See Samuel Huntington, *The Clash of Civilisations and the Remaking of World Order* (New York: Simon & Schuster, 1996).

74. Bryan Turner, *Vulnerability and Human Rights*, 62.

75. Ibid.

76. Ibid.

77. Søren Kierkegaard, *The Concept of Irony* (London: Collins, 1966), 262.

78. Alex Proyas (director), James O'Barr (comic book writer) and David J. Schow (screenplay), *The Crow* (Santa Monica, CA: Crowvision Inc., 1994).

79. Peter Beilharz, "Introduction by Peter Beilharz: Reading Zygmunt Bauman" in Peter Beilharz (ed), *The Bauman Reader* (Oxford: Blackwell,

2001), 2; see also Keith Tester, "Bauman's Irony" in Anthony Elliott (ed), *The Contemporary Bauman* (London: Routledge, 2007), 81-97.

80. Peter Beilharz, "Reading Zygmunt Bauman", 2.

81. Milan Kundera, *The Art of the Novel* (London: Faber and Faber, 1986), 134.

82. David Griner, "How 9/11 Almost Put an End to *Family Guy*", *Ad-Freak*, available at http://adweek.blogs.com/adfreak/2007/09/how-911-almost.html, 2007, retrieved on 8 September 2009.

83. Seth MacFarlane in David Griner, "How 9/11 Almost Put an End to *Family Guy*".

84. Emma Zachurski, ""American Dad": An Unpromising Start for a Rehash Pregram", *Silver Chips Online*, February 14, 2005, available at http://silverchips.mbhs.edu/story/print/4898, retrieved on 8 September 2009.

85. Seth MacFarlane in Troy Rogers, "Seth McFarlane, American Dad Interview", *UGO.com*, http://www.ugo.com/ugo/html/article/?id=17297, no date, retrieve on 8 September 2009.

86. See John Law, *After Method: Mess in Social Science Research* (London: Routledge, 2004).

87. Seth MacFarlane appearing on *Larry King Live*, 22 April 2010, *CNN*, transcript available at http://transcripts,cnn.com/TRANSCRIPTS/10040220lkl.01.html, retrieved on 28 April 2010.

88. Seth MacFarlane (creator), "It Takes a Village Idiot and I Married One", *Family Guy*, season five, episode seventeen (Los Angeles: Fuzzy Door Productions, 2007).

89. Seth MacFarlane (creator), "It Takes a Village Idiot and I Married One".

90. Jeffrey Melnick, *9/11 Culture*, 2.

91. As reproduced in Jeffrey Melnick, *9/11 Culture*, 3.

92. Sharon Pickering, *Refugees and State Crime* (Annandale, NSW: Federation Press, 2005); Kel Glare in J. Kelly, "High Flyers Can Go Jump", *Herald Sun*, 7 October 2005, 3.

93. David A. Goodman, Danny Smith (executive producers), Kara Vallow, Tom Devanney (writers), Brian Iles (director) and Seth Green (actor), audio commentaries for "Back to the Woods", *Family Guy*, Season Eight DVD [Australian version] (Moore Park, NSW: Twentieth Century Fox, 2009).

94. Neal Boushell (writer) and Seth MacFarlane (creator), "Homeland Insecurity", *American Dad*, season one, episode six (Los Angeles: 20th Century Fox Television, 2005).

95. See Luke Howie, *Terrorism, the Worker and the City: Simulations and Security in a Time of Terror* (Surrey: Gower/Ashgate, 2009), 116-119.

96. KRS-One in Jeffrey Melnick, *9/11 Culture*, 94.

97. Ward Churchill, "On the Justice of Roosting Chickens".

98. Sherman Alexie, "Flight Patterns", in *Ten Little Indians* (New York: Grove, 2003), 112.

99. My emphasis. KRS-One in Jeffrey Melnick, *9/11 Culture*, 95.

100. Jeffrey Melnick, *9/11 Culture*, 95.

101. Trey Parker, Matt Stone and Pam Brady (writers), *Team America – World Police* (Hollywood: Paramount Pictures, 2004).

102. James Gow, "Team America World Police: Down-Home Theories of Power and Peace", *Millennium – Journal of International Studies*, 2006, 34, 563.

103. Ibid, 564.

104. My emphasis. Ibid, 566.

105. "Gary" in Trey Parker, Matt Stone and Pam Brady (writers), *Team America – World Police*.

106. Ziauddin Sardar and Merryl Wyn Davies, *Why Do People Hate America?*.

107. Ibid, 63.

108. My emphasis. Ibid, 64.

109. David Swanson, "Is Best Antiwar Voice on TV Glenn Beck?", *American Chronicle*, 18 April 2010, available at http://www.americanchronicle.com/articles/view/151804, retrieved on 21 April 2010.

110. Slavoj Žižek, *First as Tragedy, Then as Farce* (London: Verso, 2009), 44.

111. Ziauddin Sardar and Merryl Wyn Davies, *Why Do People Hate America?*, 64.

112. Trey Parker, Matt Stone and Pam Brady (writers), *Team America – World Police*.

113. Ibid.

114. Ibid.

115. Ibid, 64-65.

116. Trey Parker, Matt Stone and Pam Brady (writers), *Team America – World Police*.

117. Justin Lewis, Richard Maxwell and Toby Miller, "9-11", *Television & New Media*, 3, 2: 125-131.

118. Ibid, 125.

119. Ibid.

120 Toby Miller, *Cultural Citizenship*, 81.

121.Anthony Cordesman, "Shape, Clear, Hold and Build", lecture presented to the Global Terrorism Research Centre (GTReC), 23 October 2009.

122. David Letterman, "Cool/Not Cool", available at http://www.youtube.com/watch?v=o-fOdbB3ESU, retrieved on 12 November 2009.

123. Matthew Lysiak and Corky Siemaszko, "The Enemy Within Shakes Military: Victims From Fort Hood Shooting Arrive at Dover Air Force Base", *NY Daily News*, 7 November 2009, available at http:www.nydailynews.com/news/national/2009/11/07/2009-11-07_untitled_2hood07m.html, retrieved on 15 January 2010.

124. Ibid.

125. Gustav Hasford (novel) and Stanley Kubrick (screenplay), *Full Metal Jacket* (no location: Natant, 1987).

126. James Der Derian, "Imaging Terror: Logos, Pathos and Ethos", *Third World Quarterly*, 2005, 26 (1), 26.

127. Ibid.

128. See Toby Miller, *Makeover Nation: The United States of Reinvention* (Columbus: The Ohio State University Press, 2008).

129. James Der Derian, "Imaging Terror", 37.

Chapter 7

1. Dr. John "JD" Dorian in Bill Lawrence (creator) and Mike Schwartz (writer), "My Choosiest Choice of All", *Scrubs*, episode 3.19 (Burbank, CA: Doozer, 2004).

2. Jean Baudrillard, *The Intelligence of Evil or the Lucidity Pact* (Oxford: Berg, 2005), 91.

3. TISM, "Play Mistral For Me", *TISM*, from the album *Macchiavelli and the Four Seasons* (Northcote, VIC: Shock Records).

4. *Nike* marketing campaign for LeBron James. See Street and Smith's Sports Business Daily, "Nike Rolling Out New "Witness" Campaign Around LeBron James", available at http://www.sportsbusinessdaily.com/article/112472, retrieved on 22 February 2010.

5. See Andrea Dworkin, "Pornography: The New Terrorism", *New York University Review of Law and Social Change*, 1978-1979, 8, 215-218. Where Andrea Dworkin (1978-1979) explored the terror of pornography, I will explore the pornography of terrorism. Whilst I do not intend to equate my discussion of terrorism with Dworkin's discussion of pornography, I agree with Dworkin (1978-1979: 215-216) when she wrote "Oppressed people are not subjugated or controlled by dim warnings or vague threats of harm. Their chains are not made of shadows. Oppressed people are *terrorized* – by raw violence, real violence, unspeakable and pervasive violence. Their bodies are assaulted and despoiled, according to the will of the oppressor. This violence is always accompanied by cultural assault – propaganda disguised as principle or knowledge". For Dworkin, the terrorist victimizes others with their propaganda. Perhaps oddly, among my arguments in this book is that the terrorist victimizes others with the

victims propaganda. The "cultural assault" in a time of terror is delivered by the global news media. They deliver the pornography of terrorism to witnesses (the voyeurs) in places large distances from where terrorism has occurred.

6. Sarah Kay, *Žižek: A Critical Introduction* (Cambridge: Polity, 2003), 58.

7. Slavoj Žižek, *The Parallax View* (Cambridge: The MIT Press, 2006), 17.

8. In developing this concept, I owe much to Toby Miller's book *Sportsex* (Philadelphia: Temple University Press, 2001) as well as the comments that he provided in his examination of my PhD thesis.

9. Louise Richardson, *What Terrorists Want: Understanding the Terrorist Threat* (London: John Murray, 2006), 1.

10. Walter Laqueur, "Reflections on Terrorism", *Foreign Affairs*, 1986-1987, 65, 88-89.

11. Timothy Reuter, "Lessons of Terror: A History of Warfare Against Civilians: Why It Has Always Failed and Why It Will Fail Again – Recent Books", *SAIS Review*, Summer-Fall 2002, 371.

12. Martin Ham, "Excess and Resistance in Feminised Bodies: David Cronenberg's *Videodrome* and Jean Baudrillard's *Seduction*", *Senses of Cinema*, available at http://archive.sensesofcinema.com/contents/04/30/videodrome_seduction.html, 2004, retrieved on 1 May 2009.

13. Slavoj Žižek, *Welcome to the Desert of the Real!: Five Essays on September 11 and Related Dates* (London: Verso, 2002); Jean Baudrillard, *The Spirit of Terrorism and Requiem for the Twin Towers* (London: Verso, 2002).

14. William Merrin, *Baudrillard and the Media: A Critical Introduction* (Cambridge: Polity, 2005), 38.

15. Ibid, 39.

16. Ibid.

17. Jean Baudrillard, *Seduction* (New York: St. Martin's Press, 1990), 30, 31-32.

18. Jean Baudrillard, *Simulacra and Simulation* (Ann Arbor: The University of Michigan Press, 1994), 1.

19. Jean Baudrillard, *The Gulf War Did Not Take Place* (Sydney: Power Publications, 1995).

20. The most obvious exception to this may naturally be the soldiers who were deployed to Iraq during the first Gulf War.

21. Jean Baudrillard, *The Spirit of Terrorism*.

22. Ibid, 4.

23. Ibid, 7.

24. Ibid, 18.

25 Slavoj Žižek, *Welcome to the Desert of the Real!*, 6.

26. Emphasis in original. Jean Baudrillard, *The Spirit of Terrorism*, 5.

27. Michael Ignatieff, "The Terrorist as Auteur", *The New York Times*,

14 November 2004, available at http://www.nytimes.com/2004/11/14/ movies/14TERROR.html, retrieved on 6 June 2007.

28. Ibid.

29. Daniel Ziffer, "Australian TV Viewers Too Scared to Look Away", *The Age*, 21 July 2006, 7.

30. Ibid.

31. Ibid.

32. Kim Toffoletti, *Cyborgs and Barbie Dolls: Feminism, Popular Culture and the Posthuman Body* (London: I.B. Tauris, 2007), 51.

33. Ibid.

34. Jean Baudrillard, *Seduction*, 29.

35. Akinbola Akinwumi, "The Banality of the ImMEDIAte Spectacle: Globalization, Terrorism, Radical Cultural Denigration, and the Condition of Hollowity", *International Journal of Baudrillard Studies*, 2006, 3 (1), available at http://www.ubishops.ca/baudrillardstudies/vol3_1/akinbolapf. htm, retrieved on 30 April 2009.

36. Slavoj Žižek, *Welcome to the Desert of the Real!*, 11.

37. Ibid.

38. Jean Baudrillard, "Dust Breeding", in A. Kroker and M. Kroker (eds), *CTheory*, 2001, available at http://www.ctheory.net/articles.aspx?id=293, retrieved on 7 August 2006.

39. Louise Richardson, *What Terrorists Want*, 19.

40. Jean Baudrillard, "Dust Breeding".

41. Ibid.

42. Barry Koltnow, "9/11 Families United Over Must-See Tale", *Sunday Mail*, 6 August 2006, 92.

43. And indeed the pre-9/11 world. See Walter Laqueur (1987), *The Age of Terrorism* (Boston: Little, Brown, 1987), 174-202.

44. Susanna Schrobsdorff, "Sexy or Sadistic?", *Newsweek*, 6 March 2007, available at http://www.msnbc.msn.com/id/17490782/site/newsweek/, retrieved on 8 May 2007.

45. Ibid.

46. Ibid.

47. Image available at http://www.slate.com/id/2149508, retrieved on 5 January 2010. Courtesy of *Slate*.

48. Ryan Rowe, Ed Solomon and John August (writers), *Charlie's Angels* (Los Angeles: Columbia Pictures Corporation, 2000).

49. Luc Besson (writer), *La Femme Nikita* (Neuilly sur Seine: Gaumont, 1990).

50. J. F. Lawton (writer), *Pretty Woman* (Burbank: Touchstone Pictures, 1990).

51. Mike Myers and Michael McCullers (writers), *Austin Powers: The Spy Who Shagged Me* (New York City: New Line Cinema, 1999).

52. Neal Purvis and Robert Wade (screenplay), *Casino Royale* (Los Angeles: Metro-Goldwyn-Mayer [MGM], 2008).

53. Chris Johnston, "Designer Terror-Porn Now in Vogue", *The Age*, 28 October 2006, 20.

54. Ibid.

55. Associated Press, "Nothing Sexy About Nude Scans", *The Age*, 17 May 2007, available at http://www.theage.com.au/articles/2007/05/17/1178995296128.html, retrieved on 22 May 2007.

56. Ibid.

57. Anahad O'Connor and Eric Schmitt, "Terror Attempt Seen as Man Tries to Ignite Device on Jet", *The New York Times*, 25 December 2009, available at http://www.nytimes.com/2009/12/26/us/26plane.html, retrieved on 17 February 2010.

58. Available at http://hungryblues.net/2006/10/11/abu-ghraib-usa/, retrieved on 16 February 2010, photo courtesy of Ben Greenburg; available at http://www.internationalist.org/iraqtorture0504.html, retrieved on 16 February 2010, photo courtesy of *The New Yorker* and *The Internationalist*.

59. Chris Johnston, "Designer Terror-Porn Now in Vogue", 20.

60. Susan Sontag, "What Have We Done?", *The Guardian*, 23 May 2004, G2, 3-4.

61. Slavoj Žižek, *Violence: Six Sideways Reflections* (London: Profile Books, 2008), 146.

62. Ibid.

63. Nicholas Mirzoeff, "Invisible Empire: Visual Culture, Embodied Spectacle, and Abu Ghraib", *Radical History Review*, 2006, 95, 21.

64. Jasbir Puar, *Terrorist Assemblages: Homonationalism in Queer Times* (Durham: Duke University Press, 2007); Jasbir Puar, "On Torture: Abu Ghraib", *Radical History Review*, 2005, 93, 13-38.

65. My emphasis. Jasbir Puar, "On Torture", 13.

66. Jean Baudrillard, "War Porn", *International Journal of Baudrillard Studies*, trans. By Paul A. Taylor, 2005, 2(1), available at http://www.ubishops.ca/baudrillardstudies/vol2_1/taylorpf.htm, retrieved on 1 February 2010.

67. Ibid.

68. Ibid.

69. Paul A. Taylor, "Pornographic Barbarism and the Self-Reflecting Sign", *International Journal of Baudrillard Studies*, 2007, 4(1), available at http://www.ubishops.ca/BaudrillardStudies/vol4_1/taylor.htm, retrieved on 31 January 2007.

70. Ibid.

71. Susan Sontag, "What Have We Done?".

72. Ibid.

73. Chris Johnston, "Designer Terror-Porn Now in Vogue", 20.

74. Paul Virilio, *Ground Zero* (London: Verso, 2002), 23.

75. Audrey C. Rule, "An Analysis of Dollhouse Story Themes and Related Authentic Learning Activities", *Journal of Authentic Learning*, 2(1), 61.

76. The company's fictional website set up as a promoting tool for *Dollhouse* can be found at http://www.rossumcorporation.com/.

77. Joss Whedon (creator and writer), "Ghost", *Dollhouse*, episode one, season one (Beverley Hills: Twentieth Century Fox, 2009).

78. Emily Nussbaum, "Whedon on the End of *Dollhouse*, Kinky Sex, and the Future of Online TV", *New York: NY Mag*, 3 December 2009, available at http://www.nymag.com/daily/tv/2009/12/whedon_on_the_end_of_dollhouse.html, retrieved on 16 February 2010.

79. Joss Whedon in Emily Nussbaum, "Whedon on the End of *Dollhouse*".

80. Troy Patterson, "She's Got Legs: Eliza Dushku in Joss Whedon's *Dollhouse*", *Slate*, 12 February 2009, available at http://www.slate.com/id/2211160/, retrieved on 18 February 2010.

81. Ibid.

82. Kelly West, "TV Recap: Dollhouse: True Believer", 2009, available at http://www.filmhobbit.com/television/TV-Recap-Dollhouse-True-Believer-16144.html, retrieved on 22 February 2010.

83. My emphasis. Joss Whedon (creator) and Tim Minear (writer), "True Believer", *Dollhouse*, episode five, season one (Beverley Hills: Twentieth Century Fox, 2009).

84. Ibid.

85. Robert Scheer, *The Pornography of Power: Why Defense Spending Must Be Cut* (New York: Twelve, 2008).

86. My emphasis. Ibid, xix.

87. Chris Carter (creator and writer), "The Beginning", *The X Files*, episode one, season six (Los Angeles: 20th Century Fox Television, 1998).

88. Zillah Eisenstein, *Sexual Decoys: Gender, Race and War in Imperial Democracy* (London: Zed Books, 2007), xii.

89. Ibid, 6-7.

90. Ibid, xi.

91. Ibid, 17.

92. Zillah Eisenstein, *Sexual Decoys*, 17.

93. Margaret Cho in Jeffrey Melnick, *9/11 Culture: America Under Construction* (Malden, MA: Wiley-Blackwell, 2009), 126.

94. See http://www.randomhouse.com/pantheon/graphicnovels/towers.html, retrieved on 1 March 2010; Art Spiegelman in Jeffrey Melnick, *9/11 Culture*, 126.

95. Albert M. de Plazaola, "Sexual Simulacra: Jenna Jameson, Baudrillard and Pornography", 26 November 2003, available at http:www. inter-disciplinary.net/transform/plazaola%20paper.pdf, retrieved on 3 November 2006, 2.

96. Jean Baudrillard, "Pornography of War", *Cultural Politics*, 2005, 1(1), 24.

97. Ibid.

98. Albert M. de Plazaola, "Sexual Simulacra", 1.

99. Jean Baudrillard, "Dust Breeding", in Arthur Kroker and Marilouise Kroker (eds.), *CTheory*, 2001, available at http://www.ctheory.net/articles. aspx?id=293, retrieved on 7 August 2006.

100. Nicola Smith and Jack Grimston, "European Police Probe Sex-Abuse Allegations in "Second Life"", *The Times*, 21 May 2007, available at http://www.foxnews.com/story/0,2933,273613,00.html?sPage=fnc. technology/videogaming, retrieved on 28 May 2007.

101. T. Fullerton, "You Only Live Twice", *4 Corners Broadband*, available at http://www.abc.net.au/4corners/special_eds/20070319/default_full. htm, 2007, retrieved on 28 May 2007.

102. Albert M. de Plazaola, "Sexual Simulacra", 2.

Chapter 8

1. Jack Donaghy in Tina Fey (creator) and Dave Finkel (writer), "Fireworks", *30 Rock*, season one, episode eighteen (New York: Broadway Video, 2007).

2. Judith Butler, *Precarious Life: The Powers of Mourning and Violence* (London: Verso, 2004), x.

3. Ibid, xii.

4. Ibid, 6-7.

5. Andy H, "The WTC Tragedy 1st Hand. Andy's Blog Entries 9.11.01-9.16.01", available at http://www.andyschest.com/WTC_Diary.html, retrieved on 30 April 2010.

6. Ibid.

7. Ibid.

8. Alisa Solomon, "Terror Attack", *The Village Voice*, 11 September 2001, available at http://www.villagevoice.com/2001-09-11/news/terror-attack/1, retrieved on 30 April 2010.

9. Ibid.

10. Ibid.

11. Toby Miller, "On Being Ignorant: Living in Manhattan", 2002, available at www.portalcomunicacion.com/bcn2002/n_eng/contents/11/ miller.pdf, retrieved on 1 February 2007.

12. Ibid.

13. Eliot Weinberger, *9/12: New York After* (Chicago: Prickly Paradigm Press, 2003).

14. My emphasis. Ibid, 18.

15. Noam Chomsky, *The Culture of Terrorism* (London: Pluto, 1988).

16. Edward Herman and Noam Chomsky, *Manufacturing Consent: The Political Economy of the Mass Media* (New York: Pantheon Books, 2002); see also Noam Chomsky, *The Culture of Terrorism*; Noam Chomsky and Edward Herman, *The Washington Connection and Third World Fascism* (Boston: South End Press, 1979).

17. Eliot Weinberger, *9/12: New York After*, 27.

18. Ibid.

19. Jean Baudrillard, "Dust Breeding", in Arthur Kroker and Marilouise Kroker (eds), *CTheory*, 2001, available at http://www.ctheory.net/articles. aspx?id=293, retrieved on 7 August 2006.

20. Ibid.

21. Trey Parker and Matt Stone (creators and writers), "Imaginationland", "Imaginationland: Episode II" and "Imaginationland: Episode III", *South Park*, episodes ten, eleven and twelve in season eleven (New York, Comedy Central, 2007).

22. Ibid.

23. Trey Parker and Matt Stone (creators and writers), "Imaginationland".

24. Matt Sienkiewicz and Nick Marx, "Beyond a Cutout World: Ethnic Humor and Discursive Integration in *South Park*", *Journal of Film and Video*, 2009, 61(2), available at http://muse.jhu.edu/journals/journal_of_film_ and_video/v061/61.2.sienkiewicz.html, retrieved on 23 March 2010.

25. Ibid.

26. Trey Parker and Matt Stone (creators and writers), "Imaginationland".

27. Daniel Keyes, "Canada and Saddam in *South Park*: Aboot Allah", in Leslie Stratyner and James R. Keller (eds.), *The Deep End of South Park: Critical Essays on Television's Shocking Cartoon Series* (Jefferson, NC: McFarland & Company, 2009), 152-153.

28. Trey Parker and Matt Stone (creators and writers), "Imaginationland".

29. Jean Baudrillard, *The Spirit of Terrorism and Requiem for the Twin Towers* (London: Verso, 2002); Slavoj Žižek, *Welcome to the Desert of the Real! Five Essays on September 11 and Related Dates* (London: Verso, 2002).

30. Lee Ben Clarke, *Worst Cases: Terror and Catastrophe in the Popular Imagination* (Chicago: University of Chicago Press, 2006), ix.

31. Gerd Gigerenzer in Dan Gardner, *Risk: The Science and Politics of Fear* (Melbourne: Scribe, 2008), 3-4.

32. Ibid, x.

33. Ibid.

34. Eliot Weinberger, *9/12: New York After*, 27-28.

35. Guy Debord, *The Society of the Spectacle* (Detroit: Black & Red, 1987).

36. Julia Kristeva in John Lechte, "The Imaginary and the Spectacle: Kristeva's View", in John Lechte and Maria Margaroni (eds.), *Julia Kristeva: Live Theory* (London: Continuum, 2005), 116-117.

37. John Lechte, "The Imaginary and the Spectacle", 116-117.

38. Slavoj Žižek, *On Belief* (London: Routledge, 2001), 47.

39. Julia Kristeva in John Lechte, "The Imaginary and the Spectacle", 117.

40. Andy H, "The WTC Tragedy 1st Hand".

41. Alan Wolfe, "The Home Front: American Society Responds to the New War", in James F. Hoge, Jr. and Gideon Rose (eds.), *How Did This Happen?: Terrorism and the New War* (New York: Public Affairs, 2001), 283.

Bibliography

Abrams, J.J. (creator). *Alias*. Burbank, CA: Touchstone Television, 2001.

Agamben, Georgio. *Homo Sacer: Sovereign Power and Bare Life*, trans. by D. Heller-Roazen. Stanford, CA: Stanford University Press, 1998.

Akinwumi, Akinbola. "The Banality of the ImMEDIAte Spectacle: Globalization, Terrorism, Radical Cultural Denigration, and the Condition of Hollowity", *International Journal of Baudrillard Studies*, 2006, 3(1), available at http://www.ubishops.ca/baudrillardstudies/vol3_1/akinbolapf.htm, retrieved on 30 April 2009.

Alexander, Jeffrey C.; Eyerman, Ron; Giesen, Bernhard. *Cultural Trauma and Collective Identity*. Berkeley: University of California Press, 2004.

Alexander, Jeffrey C.; Eyerman, Ron; Giesen, Bernhard; Smelser, Neil J. and Sztrompka, Piotr. *Cultural Trauma*. Berkeley: University of California Press, 2000.

Alexie, Sherman. *Ten Little Indians*. New York: Grove, 2003.

Andrejevic, Mark. "The Body, Torture, and the Decline of Symbolic Efficiency", *Politics and Culture*, no date, available at http://aspen.conncoll.edu/politicsandculture/page.cfm?key=538, retrieved on 20 January 2010.

Andy H. "The WTC Tragedy 1st Hand. Andy's Blog Entries 9.11.01-9.16.01", available at http://www.andyschest.com/WTC_Diary.html, retrieved on 30 April 2010.

Associated Press. "Nothing Sexy About Nude Scans", *The Age*, 17 May 2007, available at http://www.theage.com.au/articles/2007/05/17/1178895296128.html, retrieved on 22 May 2007.

Associated Press. "Barack Obama Stops Wearing American Flag Lapel Pin", *Fox News*, 4 October 2007, available at http://www.foxnews.com/printer_friendly_story/0,3566,299439,00.html, retrieved on 11 November 2008.

Atwater, Tony. "Network Evening News Coverage of the TWA Hostage Crisis", in Yonah Alexander and Richard Latter (eds.), *Terrorism & the Media: Dilemmas for Government, Journalists & the Public*. Washington: Brassey's, 1990, 85-92.

Australian Human Right Commission, "Fact Sheet: Australian Muslims", available at http://www.hreoc.gov.au/racial_discrimination/isma/consultations/facts/fact_muslim.html, retrieved on 3 May 2010.

Avery, Dylan (writer), *Loose Change 9/11: An American Coup*. Location details unavailable: Louder Than Words, 2005.

Ayloush, Hussam. Letter to Matt Groening, the creator and director of *The Simpsons*, 3 December 2008, available at http://cair-california.org/images/stories/thank_you_letter_-_matt_groening.pdf, retrieved on 17 September 2009.

Barlow, Aaron. *The Rise of the Blogosphere*. Westport, Conn: Praeger, 2007.

Barthes, Roland. *Image – Music – Text*. New York: Hill and Wang, 1978.

Bartosiewicz, Petra. "Experts in Terror", *The Nation*, 17 January 2008, available at http://www.thenation.com/doc/20080204/bartosiewicz/print, retrieved on 5 March 2010.

Baudrillard, Jean. *Seduction*. New York: St. Martin's Press, 1990.

Baudrillard, Jean. *Simulacra and Simulation*. Ann Arbor: The University of Michigan Press, 1994.

Baudrillard, Jean. *The Gulf War Did Not Take Place*. Sydney: Power Publications, 1995.

Baudrillard, Jean. "Dust Breeding", in A. Kroker and M. Kroker (eds), *CTheory*, 2001, available at http://www.ctheory.net/articles.aspx?id=293, retrieved on 7 August 2006.

Baudrillard, Jean. *The Spirit of Terrorism and Requiem for the Twin Towers*. London: Verso, 2002.

Baudrillard, Jean. *The Intelligence of Evil or the Lucidity Pact*. Oxford: Berg, 2005.

Baudrillard, Jean. "War Porn", *International Journal of Baudrillard Studies*, trans. By Paul A. Taylor, 2005, 2(1), available at http://www.ubishops.ca/baudrillardstudies/vol2_1/taylorpf.htm, retrieved on 1 February 2010.

Baudrillard, Jean. "Pornography of War", *Cultural Politics*, 2005, 1(1), 23-24.

Bauman, Zygmunt. *Liquid Life*. Cambridge: Polity, 2005.

Bauman, Zygmunt. *Liquid Fear*. Cambridge: Polity, 2006.

Bauman, Zygmunt. *Does Ethics Have a Chance in a World of Consumers?* Cambridge: Harvard University Press, 2008.

Baumgartner, Jody and Morris, Jonathan S. "*The Daily Show* Effect: Candidate Evaluations, Efficacy, and American Youth", *American Politics Research*, 34(3), 341-367.

Barnett, Michael. "From Me to We ... and Back Again: Returning to Business as Usual", *Journal of Management Inquiry*, 2002, 11(3), 249-252.

BBC News. "Toll Climbs in Egyptian Attacks", *BBC News*, 23 July 2005, available at http://news.bbc.co.uk/2/hi/middle_east/4709491.stm, retrieved on 15 March 2010.

BBC News. "Gunmen Shoot Sri Lanka Cricketers", *BBC News*, 3 March 2009, available at http://news.bbc.co.uk/go/pr/fr/-/2/hi/south_asia/7920260. stm, retrieved on 8 May 2009.

BBC News. "US Marks Seventh 9/11 Anniversary", *BBC News*, 11 September 2008, available at http://news.bbc.co.uk/2/hi/americas/7609636.stm, retrieved on 19 August 2009.

Beck, Ulrich and Beck-Gernsheim, Elizabeth. *Individualization: Institutionalized Individualism and Its Social and Political Consequences*. London: Sage, 2002.

Beilharz, Peter. "Introduction by Peter Beilharz: Reading Zygmunt Bauman" in Peter Beilharz (ed). *The Bauman Reader*. Oxford: Blackwell, 2001, 1-17.

Berg, Rick. "Losing Vietnam: Covering the War in an Age of Technology", *Cultural Critique*, 1986, 3, Spring, 92-125.

Besson, Luc (writer). *La Femme Nikita*. Neuilly sur Seine: Gaumont, 1990.

Boushell, Neal (writer) and MacFarlane, Seth (creator). "Homeland Insecurity", *American Dad*, season one, episode six. Los Angeles: 20th Century Fox Television, 2005.

Burloff, Andrea and McLoughlin, John (writers). *World Trade Center*. Hollywood, CA: Paramount Pictures, 2006.

Butler, Judith. *Precarious Life: The Powers of Mourning and Violence*. London: Verso, 2004.

Button, James. "They Swear to Save Lives", *The Age*, 4 July 2007, 1.

Callaghan, Dylan. "Those Were the Days", *Writers Guild of America*, available from http://www.wga.org/content/default.aspx?id=3118, 2009, retrieved on 22 April 2009.

Campbell, Perri and Kelly, Peter. "'Explosions and Examinations': Growing Up Female in Post-Saddam Iraq", *Journal of Youth Studies*, 2009, 12(1), 21-38.

Carter, Chris (creator and writer). "The Beginning", *The X Files*, episode one, season six. Los Angeles: 20th Century Fox Television, 1998.

Carter, Chris and Spotnitz, Frank (writers). *The X Files: Fight the Future*. Los Angeles: Twentieth Century Fox, 1998.

Caruth, Cathy (ed). *Trauma: Explorations in Memory*. Baltimore: Johns Hopkins University Press, 1995.

Caruth, Cathy. *Unclaimed Experience: Trauma, Narrative, and History*. Baltimore: Johns Hopkins University Press, 1996.

Casey, Jim. ""All This Has Happened Before": Repetition, Reimagination, and Eternal Return", in Tiffany Potter and C.W. Marshall (eds.). *Cylons in America: Critical Studies in* Battlestar Galactica. New York: Continuum, 2008, 237-250.

Cashmore, Ellis. *Celebrity/Culture*. Abingdon: Routledge, 2006.

Chauncey Billups. "Celebrity Obsession and Terrorism", available at http://blogcritics.org/scitech/article/celebrity-obsession-and-terrorism/, 2005, retrieved on 5 March 2010.

Chomsky, Noam and Herman, Edward. *The Washington Connection and Third World Fascism*. Boston: South End Press, 1979.

Chomsky, Noam. *The Culture of Terrorism*. Boston: South End Press, 1988.

Chomsky, Noam. *September 11*. Crows Nest, NSW: Allen and Unwin, 2001.

Chomsky, Noam (interviewed by Dimitriadis Epaminondas). "On the War Against Terrorism and Related Issues", 3 July 2002, available at http://www.chomsky.info/interviews/20020703.htm, retrieved on 30 March 2008.

Churchill, Ward. ""Some People Push Back": On the Justice of Roosting Chickens", available at http://www.kersplebedeb.com/mystuff/s11/churchill.html, 2003, retrieved on 3 July 2008.

Churchill, Ward. *On the Justice of Roosting Chickens: Reflections on the Consequences of U.S. Imperial Arrogance and Criminality*. Oakland, CA: AK Press, 2003.

Clarke, Lee Ben. *Worst Cases: Terror and Catastrophe in the Popular Imagination*. Chicago: University of Chicago Press, 2006.

Clymer, Jeffory. *America's Culture of Terrorism: Violence, Capitalism and the Written Word*. Chapel Hill: University of North Carolina Press, 2003.

CNN, "September 11 – A Memorial", *CNN.com*, 2002, available at http://www.cnn.com/SPECIALS/2001/memorial/people/2144.html, accessed on 10 July 2008.

Cochran, Robert and Surnow, Joel (creators). *24*. Beverly Hills, CA: Imagine Entertainment, 2001.

Colen, Alexandra. "Paris Hilton Terrorism", *The Brussels Journal*, 2008, available http://www.brusselsjournal.com/node/3673, retrieved on 29 May 2009.

Conrad, Joseph. *The Secret Agent*. London, Vintage Books, [1920] 2007.

Coogan, Tim Pat. *The I.R.A.* London: Harper Collins, 2000.

Coorey, Phillip. "Increased Terror Risk From Within", *The Sydney Morning Herald*, 23 February 2010, 1.

Cordesman, Anthony. "Shape, Clear, Hold and Build", lecture presented to the Global Terrorism Research Centre (GTReC), 23 October 2009.

Cornish, Paul. "The Age of "Celebrity Terrorism"", *BBC News*, 30 November 2008, available at http://news.bbc.co.uk/go/pr/fr/-/2/hi/south_asia/7755684.stm, retrieved on 23 July 2009.

Crane, David and Kauffman, Marta (creators). *Friends* [television series 1994-2004]. Burbank: Warner Brothers, 1994.

Crane, David and Kauffman, Marta (creators). "The One After "I Do"", *Friends*, season eight, episode one. Burbank: Warner Brothers Studios, 2001.

Crane, David and Kauffman, Marta (creators). "The One Where Rachel Tells", *Friends*, season eight, episode three. Burbank: Warner Brothers Studios, 2001.

Crane, David and Kauffman, Marta (creators). "The One Where Joey Dates Rachel", season eight, episode twelve. Burbank: Warner Brothers Studios, 2001.

Crawford, Carly and Hudson, Fiona. "Aussie Swoop as Police Believe They Have Cracked a Ring of ... TERROR DOCTORS", *Herald Sun*, 4 July 2007, 1.

Debord, Guy. *The Society of the Spectacle*. Detroit: Black & Red, 1987.

de Plazaola, Albert M. "Sexual Simulacra: Jenna Jameson, Baudrillard and Pornography", 26 November 2003, available at http:www.interdisciplinary.net/transform/plazaola%20paper.pdf, retrieved on 3 November 2006.

Der Derian, James. "Imaging Terror: Logos, Pathos and Ethos", *Third World Quarterly*, 2005, 26(1), 23-37.

Derrickson, Scott (director); Scarpa, David (screenplay) and North, Edmund H. (screenplay, 1951). *The Day The Earth Stood Still*. Los Angeles: Twentieth Century Fox, 2008.

Dick Destiny. "Celebrity Terrorism Expert", *Dick Destiny*, 28 August 2009, available at http://www.dickdestiny.com/blog/2009/08/celebrity-terrorism-expert-always-there.html, retrieved on 5 March 2010.

Domiciliphile. "The Age of "Celebrity Terrorism"", 30 November 2008, available at http://digg.com/world_news/The_age_of_celebrity_terrorism, retrieved on 23 July 2009.

Dudley, Michael. "*Battlestar Galactica*: Immersion Therapy for Post 9/11 World", available at http://www.alternet.org/module/printversion/133419, 2009, retrieved on 14 January 2010.

Dworkin, Andrea. "Pornography: The New Terrorism", *New York University Review of Law and Social Change*, 1978-1979, 8, 215-218.

Edkins, Jennifer. "Forget Trauma? Response to September 11", *International Relations*, 2002, 16(2), 243-256.

Eisenstein, Zillah. *Sexual Decoys: Gender, Race and War in Imperial Democracy*. London: Zed Books, 2007.

Elliott, Anthony. *Concepts of the Self*, 2nd edn. Cambridge: Polity, 2007.

Faludi, Susan. *The Terror Dream: Fear and Fantasy in Post-9/11 America*. Melbourne: Scribe, 2008.

Fey, Tina (creator) and Finkel, Dave (writer). "Fireworks", *30 Rock*, season one, episode eighteen. New York: Broadway Video, 2007.

Freeman, Mark. "Data are Everywhere: Narrative Criticism in the Literature of Experience", in Colette Daiute and Cynthia Lightfoot (eds). *Narrative Analysis: Studying the Development of Individuals in Society*. Thousand Oaks: Sage, 2004, 63-82.

Freyd, Jenny. "In the Wake of Terrorist Attack, Hatred May Mask Fear", *Analyses of Social Issues and Public Policy*, 2002, 2(1), 5-8.

Friedland, Nehemia and Merari, Ariel. "The Psychological Impact of Terrorism: A Double-edged Sword", *Political Psychology*, 1985, 6(4), 591-604.

Fromkin, D. "The Strategy of Terrorism", *Foreign Affairs*, 53(4), 684-685.

Fromm, Erich. *The Sane Society*. London: Routledge, [1956] 2008.

Fullerton, T. "You Only Live Twice", 4 *Corners Broadband*, available at http://www.abc.net.au/4corners/special_eds/20070319/default_full.htm, 2007, retrieved on 28 May 2007.

Fusar-Poli, Paolo; Howes, Oliver; Valmaggia, Lucia and McGuire, Philip. "'Truman' Signs and Vulnerability to Psychosis", *The British Journal of Psychiatry*, 2008, 193, 168.

Gardner, Dan. *Risk: The Science and Politics of Fear*. Melbourne: Scribe, 2008.

Gay, Jason. "Dave at Peace: The Rolling Stone Interview", *Rollingstone.com*, available at http://www.rollingstone.com/news/story/22791344/dave_at_peace_the_rolling_stone_interview/print, retrieved on 7 September 2009.

Giroux, Henry. *Beyond the Spectacle of Terrorism: Global Uncertainty and the Challenge of the New Media*. Boulder: Paradigm, 2006.

Goodman, David A.; Smith, Danny (executive producers); Vallow, Kara; Devanney, Tom (writers); Iles, Brian (director) and Green, Seth (actor). Audio commentaries for "Back to the Woods", *Family Guy*, season Eight DVD [Australian version]. Moore Park, NSW: Twentieth Century Fox, 2009.

Gorman, Bill. "*Battlestar Galactica* Finale Blasts Away the Competition", 2009, available at http://tvbythenumbers.com/2009/03/24/battlestar-galactica-finale-blasts-away-the-competition/15054, retrieved on 18 January 2010.

Gow, James. "Team America World Police: Down-Home Theories of Power and Peace", *Millennium – Journal of International Studies*, 2006, 34, 563-568.

Grabiak, Marita and Moore, Ronald D. "Water", *Battlestar Galactica*, episode two, season one. Hollywood: Universal Studios, 2004.

Greengrass, Paul (writer and creator). *United 93*. Universal City, CA: Universal Pictures, 2006.

Gregory, Peter and Hunter, Thomas. "Counter-terrorism Raids Across Melbourne", *The Age*, 4 August 2009, http://www.theage.com.au/national/counterterrorism-raids-across-melbourne-20090804-e7i5.html, retrieved on 17 March 2010.

Greene, Eric. "The Mirror Frakked: Reflections on *Battlestar Galactica*", in Richard Hatch (ed.), *So Say We All: An Unauthorized Collection of*

Thoughts and Opinions on Battlestar Galactica. Dallas: Benbella Books, 2006, 5-22.

Greenwald, Robert. *Outfoxed: Rupert Murdoch's War on Journalism*. Columbia, SC: Carolina Productions, 2004.

Griner, David. "How 9/11 Almost Put an End to *Family Guy*", *AdFreak*, available at http://adweek.blogs.com/adfreak/2007/09/how-911-almost.html, 2007, retrieved on 8 September 2009.

Grosz, Elizabeth. *Space, Time and Perversion: The Politics of Bodies*. St Leonards: Allen & Unwin, 1995.

Grosz, Elizabeth. *Architecture From the Outside: Essays on Virtual and Real Space*. Cambridge: The MIT Press, 2001.

Haaretz. "Muslim Leader Threatens to Kill Paul McCartney Over Israel Gig", *Haaretz.com*, available at http://www.haaretz.com/hasen/spages/1020917.html, 2008, retrieved on 8 June 2009.

Ham, Martin. "Excess and Resistance in Feminised Bodies: David Cronenberg's *Videodrome* and Jean Baudrillard's *Seduction*", *Senses of Cinema*, available at http://archive.sensesofcinema.com/contents/04/30/videodrome_seduction.html, 2004, retrieved on 1 May 2009.

Haraway, Donna. *Simians, Cyborgs and Women: The Reinvention of Nature*. London: Free Association, 1991.

Haraway, Donna. *Modest_Witness@Second_Millenium.FemaleMan©_Meets_OncoMouse™: Feminism and Technoscience*. New York: Routledge, 1997.

Haraway, Donna (interviewed by Thyrza Nichols Goodeve). *How Like a Leaf: An Interview with Thyrza Nichols Goodeve*. New York: Routledge, 2000.

Hasford, Gustav (novel) and Kubrick, Gustav (screenplay). *Full Metal Jacket*. No location: Natant, 1987.

Heidegger, Martin. *Poetry, Language, Thought*. New York: Perennial Classics, 1971.

Herald Sun. "Four Arrests in Terror Swoop", *Herald Sun*, 4 August 2009.

Herman, Edward and Chomsky, Noam. *Manufacturing Consent: The Political Economy of the Mass Media*. New York: Pantheon Books, 2002.

Herman, Judith. *Trauma and Recovery*. New York: Basic Books, 1992.

Hirst, Rob. *Willie's Bar & Grill: A Rock 'n' Roll Tour of North America in the Age of Terror*. Sydney: Picador, 2003.

Horgan, John. *The Psychology of Terrorism*. London: Routledge, 2005.

Howie, Luke. *Terrorsex: Witnesses and the Reanimation of 9/11 as Image-event, Commodity and Pornography*. Unpublished PhD thesis, Melbourne, Monash University, January 2008.

Howie, Luke. *Terrorism, the Worker and the City: Simulations and Security in a Time of Terror*. Surrey, UK: Gower/Ashgate, 2009.

Howie, Luke. "Representing Terrorism: Reanimating Post-9/11 New York

City", *International Journal of Žižek Studies*, 2009, 3(3), available at http://zizekstudies.org/index.php/ijzs/issue/view/15, retrieved on 5 January 2010.

Howie, Luke. "Australia's History of Terrorism: Institutionalized Discrimination and the Response of the Mob", in Sean Brawley (ed), *Doomed To Repeat? Terrorism and the Lessons of History*. Washington D.C.: New Academia, 2009, 251-276.

Hunter, Thomas. "Counter-terrorism Raids Across Melbourne", *Brisbane Times*, 4 August 2009, retrieved on http://www.brisbanetimes.com.au/national/counterterrorism-raids-across-melbourne-20090804-e7iu.html, retrieved on 17 March 2010.

Huntington, Samuel. *The Clash of Civilisations and the Remaking of World Order*. New York: Simon & Schuster, 1996.

Ignatieff, Michael. "The Terrorist as Auteur", *The New York Times*, 14 November 2004, available at http://www.nytimes.com/2004/11/14/movies/14TERROR.html, retrieved on 6 June 2007.

IMDb. "Simpsons Creator Defends Muslim Plot", available at http://www.imdb.com/news/ni0645713/, retrieved on 18 September 2009.

Insurge. "Speculator", from the album *Power to the Poison People*. Crows Nest, NSW: Warner Music Australia, 1996.

Insurge. "51%", from the album *Power to the Poison People*. Crows Nest, NSW: Warner Music Australia, 1996.

Irco. "The Age of "Celebrity Terrorism"", 1 December 2008, available at http://digg.com/world_news/The_age_of_celebrity_terrorism, retrieved on 23 July 2009.

Jenkins, Brian. "The Future Course of International Terrorism", in Paul Wilkinson and Alasdair Stewart (eds), *Contemporary Research on Terrorism*. Aberdeen: Aberdeen University Press, 1987, 581-589.

Jenkins, Simon. "Indiscriminate Slaughter From the Air is a Barbarism that must be Abolished", *The Guardian*, 16 January 2009, available at http://www.guardian.co.uk/commentisfree/2009/jan/16/gaza-aerial-bombing-david-miliband/print, retrieved on 7 January 2010.

Jhally, Sut and Earp, Jeremy (eds.). *Hijacking Catastrophe: 9/11, Fear and the Selling of American Empire*. Northampton: Olive Branch Press, 2004.

Johnston, Chris. "Designer Terror-Porn Now in Vogue", *The Age*, 28 October 2006, 20.

Johnson, David Kyle. ""A Story that is Told Again and Again, and Again": Recurrence, Providence and Freedom", in Jason T. Eberl (ed.) *Battlestar Galactica and Philosophy: Knowledge Here Begins Out There*. Malden, MA: Blackwell, 2008, 181-191.

Johnson-Lewis, Erika. "Torture, Terrorism, and Other Aspects of Human Nature", in Tiffany Potter and C.W. Marshall (eds.). *Cylons in America:*

Critical Studies in Battlestar Galactica. New York: Continuum, 2008, 327-39.

Kay, Sarah. *Žižek: A Critical Introduction*. Cambridge: Polity, 2003.

Kellner, Douglas. *Media Spectacle and the Crisis of Democracy: Terrorism, War and Election Battles*. London: Paradigm, 2005.

Kelly, J. "High Flyers Can Go Jump", *Herald Sun*, 7 October 2005, 3.

Keyes, Daniel. "Canada and Saddam in *South Park*: Aboot Allah", in Leslie Stratyner and James R. Keller (eds.). *The Deep End of South Park: Critical Essays on Television's Shocking Cartoon Series*. Jefferson, NC: McFarland & Company, 2009, 139-156.

Kierkegaard, Søren. *The Concept of Irony*. London: Collins, 1966.

Kierkegaard, Søren. *Fear and Trembling/Repetition: Kierkegaard's Writings, VI*, trans. by H. V. Hong and E. H. Hong. Princeton, NJ: Princeton University Press, 1983.

Kiernan, Denise and D'Agnese, Joseph. *The Official CTU Operations Manual*. Philadelphia: Quirk Books, 2007.

Kilcullen, David. *The Accidental Guerilla: Fighting Small Wars in the Midst of a Big One*. Melbourne: Scribe, 2009.

Koltnow, Barry. "9/11 Families United Over Must-See Tale", *Sunday Mail*, 6 August 2006, 92.

Kristeva, Julia. "Stabat Mater", *Poetics Today*, 1985, 6(1-2), 133-152.

Kruse, Nancy (director) and Wilmore, Marc (writer), "Midnight RX", *The Simpsons*, episode 1606, available at http://www.wtso.net/movie/208-The_Simpsons_1606_Midnight_Rx.html, retrieved on 18 September 2009.

Kubiak, Anthony. *Stages of Terror: Terrorism, Ideology, and Coercion as Theatre History*. Bloomington: Indiana University Press, 1991.

Kuipers, Giselinde. ""Where Was King Kong When We Needed Him?" Public Discourse, Digital Disaster Jokes, and the Functions of Laughter After 9/11", *The Journal of American Culture*, 2005, 28(1), 70-84.

Kundera, Milan. *The Art of the Novel*. London: Faber and Faber, 1986.

Laqueur, Walter. "Reflections on Terrorism", *Foreign Affairs*, 1986-1987, 65, 86-100.

Laqueur, Walter. *The Age of Terrorism*. Boston: Little, Brown and Company, 1987.

Laqueur, Walter. *The New Terrorism: Fanaticism and the Arms of Mass Destruction*. London: Phoenix Press, 1999.

Laqueur, Walter. *No End to War: Terrorism in the Twenty-First Century*. New York: Continuum, 2003.

Larsen, Dana. "Tal Host Tokers", *Cannabis Culture: Marijuana Magazine*, 25 May 2009, available at http://www.cannabisculture.com/articles/4284.html, retrieved on 10 November 2009.

Law, John. *After Method: Mess In Social Science Research*. London: Routledge, 2004.

Lawrence, Bill (creator) and Schwartz, Mike (writer). "My Choosiest Choice of All", *Scrubs*, episode 3.19. Burbank, CA: Doozer, 2004.

Lawton, J. F. (writer). *Pretty Woman*. Burbank: Touchstone Pictures, 1990.

Lechte, John. "The Imaginary and the Spectacle: Kristeva's View", in John Lechte and Maria Margaroni (eds.). *Julia Kristeva: Live Theory*. London: Continuum, 2005, 116-142.

Lee, Carol D.; Rosenfeld, Erica; Mendenhall, Ruby; Rivers, Ama and Tynes, Brendesha. "Cultural Modeling as a Frame for Narrative Analysis", in Colette Daiute and Cynthia Lightfoot (eds). *Narrative Analysis: Studying the Development of Individuals in Society*. Thousand Oaks: Sage, 2004, 39-62.

Letterman, David. *Late Show*, 17 September 2001, available at http://video.google.com.au/videosearch?q=Letterman+post-9%2F11&hl=en&emb=0&aq=f#, retrieved on 7 May 2009.

Letterman, David. "Cool/Not Cool", available at http://www.youtube.com/watch?v=o-fOdbB3ESU, retrieved on 12 November 2009.

Lewis, Justin; Maxwell, Richard and Miller, Toby. "9-11", *Television & New Media*, 2002, 3(2), 125-131.

Liman, Doug and Greengrass, Paul. *The Bourne Trilogy: The Bourne Identity, The Bourne Supremacy, The Bourne Ultimatum*. Hollywood: Universal Studios, 2002-2007.

Lule, Jack. "Sacrifice and the Body on the Tarmac: Symbolic Significance of U.S News About a Terrorist Victim", in Yonah Alexander and Robert Picard (eds.), *In the Camera's Eye: News Coverage of Terrorist Events*. Washington: Brassey's, 1991, 30-45.

Lysiak, Matthew and Siemaszko, Corky. "The Enemy Within Shakes Military: Victims From Fort Hood Shooting Arrive at Dover Air Force Base", *New York Daily News*, 7 November 2009, available at http://www.nydailynews.com/news/national/2009/11/07/2009-11-07_untitled__2hood07m.html, retrieved on 9 November 2009.

MacFarlane, Seth (creator). "It Takes a Village Idiot and I Married One", *Family Guy*, season five, episode seventeen. Los Angeles: Fuzzy Door Productions, 2007.

MacFarlane, Seth. Appearing on *Larry King Live*, 22 April 2010, CNN, transcript available at http://transcripts,cnn.com/TRANSCRIPTS/10040220lkl.01.html, retrieved on 28 April 2010.

McKay, Hollie. "Is Singer Heather Schmid Being Targeted by Terrorists?", *Fox News*, 18 March 2009, available at http://www.foxnews.com/story/0,2933,509649,00.html, retrieved on 27 July 2009.

McNair, Brian. *Cultural Chaos: Journalism, News, and Power in a Globalised World*. New York: Routledge, 2006.

Manning, Peter. *Us and Them: A Journalist's Investigation of Media, Muslims and the Middle East*. Milsons Point, NSW: Random House Australia, 2006.

Martel, Ned. "Television Review; The Cylons are Back and Humanity is in Deep Trouble", *New York Times*, 8 December 2003, available at http://www.nytimes.com/2003/12/08/arts/television-review-the-cylons-are-back-and-humanity-is-in-deep-trouble.html, retrieved on 11 December 2009.

Melançon, Louis. "Secrets and Lies: Balancing Security and Democracy in the Colonial Fleet", in Josef Steiff and Tristan D. Tamplin (eds.), *Battlestar Galactica and Philosophy: Mission Accomplished or Mission Frakked Up?* Chicago: Open Court, 2008, 211-220.

Melnick, Jeffrey. *9/11 Culture: America Under Construction*. Malden, MA: John Wiley & Sons, 2009.

Merrin, William. *Baudrillard and the Media: A Critical Introduction*. Cambridge: Polity, 2005.

Miller, David and Mills, Tom. "The Terror Experts and the Mainstream Media: The Expert Nexus and its Dominance in the News Media", *Critical Studies on Terrorism*, 2009, 2(3), 414-437.

Miller, Toby. *Sportsex*. Philadelphia: Temple University Press, 2002.

Miller, Toby. "On Being Ignorant: Living in Manhattan", 2002, available at www.portalcomunicacion.com/bcn2002/n_eng/contents/11/miller.pdf, retrieved on 1 February 2007.

Miller, Toby. *Cultural Citizenship: Cosmopolitanism, Consumerism, and Television in a Neoliberal Age*. Philadelphia: Temple University Press, 2007.

Miller, Toby. *Makeover Nation: The United States of Reinvention*. Columbus: The Ohio State University Press, 2008.

Mirzoeff, Nicholas. "Invisible Empire: Visual Culture, Embodied Spectacle, and Abu Ghraib", *Radical History Review*, 2006, 95, 21-44.

Moore, Steven Dean (director) and Wilmore, Marc (writer). "Mypods and Boomsticks", *The Simpsons*, episode 2007, available at http://www.wtso.net/movie/440-2007_Mypods_and_Boomsticks.html, retrieved on 17 September 2009.

Moore, Michael (writer). *Fahrenheit 9/11*. Location details unavailable: Fellowship Adventure Group, 2004.

Moore, Ronald D. and James, Christopher (writers). *Battlestar Galactica*. Hollywood: Universal Studios, 2004.

Mueller, John. *Overblown: How Politicians and the Terrorism Industry Inflate National Security Threats, and Why We Believe Them*. New York: Free Press, 2006.

Myers, Mike and McCullers, Michael (writers). *Austin Powers: The Spy Who Shagged Me*. New York City: New Line Cinema, 1999.

Nacos, Brigitte. *Terrorism & the Media: From the Iran Hostage Crisis to the Oklahoma City Bombing*. New York: Columbia University Press, 1994.

Nacos, Brigitte. *Mass-Mediated Terrorism: The Central Role of the Media in Terrorism and Counterterrorism*. Lanham: Rowman and Littlefield Publishers, 2002.

Neal, Arthur G. *National Trauma and Collective Memory*. Armonk: M.E. Sharpe, 1998.

Neumeier, Edward (writer of screenplay) and Heinlein, Robert A. (writer of book). *Starship Troopers*. Culver City, CA: TriStar Pictures, 1997.

Niven, David; Lichter, S. Robert and Amundson, Daniel. "The Political Content of Late Night Comedy", *The Harvard International Journal of Press/Politics*, 8(3), 2003, 118-133.

Norman, Tony. "The Hilarious Dangerous World of Dave Chappelle", *Post-Gazette*, 2004, available at http://www.post-gazette.com/columnists/20040127normanp5.asp, retrieved on 22 January 2010.

Nussbaum, Emily. "Whedon on the End of *Dollhouse*, Kinky Sex, and the Future of Online TV", *New York: NY Mag*, 3 December 2009, available at http://www.nymag.com/daily/tv/2009/12/whedon_on_the_end_of_dollhouse.html, retrieved on 16 February 2010.

Oakley, Bill; Weinstein, Josh and Reardon, Jim. "The City of New York vs. Homer Simpson", *The Simpsons* – audio commentary special feature of season nine, episode one. Moore Park, NSW: Twentieth Century Fox, 2007.

O'Connor, Anahad and Schmitt, Eric. "Terror Attempt Seen as Man Tries to Ignite Device on Jet", *The New York Times*, 25 December 2009, available at http://www.nytimes.com/2009/12/26/us/26plane.html, retrieved on 17 February 2010.

Ott, Brian L. "(Re)Framing Fear: Equipment for Living in a Post-9/11 World", in Tiffany Potter and C.W. Marshall (eds.). *Cylons in America: Critical Studies in* Battlestar Galactica. New York: Continuum, 2008, 13-26.

Parker, Trey; Stone, Matt and Brady, Pam (writers). *Team America – World Police*. Hollywood: Paramount Pictures, 2004.

Parker, Trey and Stone, Matt (creators and writers). "Imaginationland", "Imaginationland: Episode II" and "Imaginationland: Episode III", *South Park*, episodes ten, eleven and twelve in season eleven. New York, Comedy Central, 2007.

Patterson, Troy. "She's Got Legs: Eliza Dushku in Joss Whedon's *Dollhouse*", *Slate*, 12 February 2009, available at http://www.slate.com/id/2211160/, retrieved on 18 February 2010.

Paust, Jordan. "A Definitional Focus", in Yonah Alexander and Seymour Finger (eds.), *Terrorism: Interdisciplinary Perspectives*. New York: John Jay Press, 1977, 18-29.

Pemberton, Greg. "Bombs Aimed at Heart of Democracy", *The Australian*, 4 July 2007, 14.

Perrin, Ben. "Gauntlet Opinions – Celebrity Terrorism", *The Gauntlet*, 11 September 1998, available at http://thegauntlet.ca/a/story/4184, retrieved on 15 March 2010.

Pickering, Sharon. *Refugees and State Crime*. Annandale, NSW: Federation Press, 2005.

Pinedo, Isabel. "Playing With Fire Without Getting Burned: Blowback Re-imagined", in Josef Steiff and Tristan D. Tamplin (eds.), Battlestar Galactica *and Philosophy: Mission Accomplished Or Mission Frakked Up?* Chicago: Open Court, 2008, 173-184.

Pinsky, Robert. "Impossible to Tell", in *The Figured Wheel: New and Collected Poems, 1966-1996*. New York: Farrar, Straus and Giroux, 1996. Poem available at http://www.ibiblio.org/ipa/poems/pinsky/impossible_to_tell.php, retrieved on 11 January 2010.

Pipes, Daniel. "Sheik Obama and His Two Wars", available at http://www.danielpipes.org/, 2009, retrieved 3 January 2010.

Plotnik, Rod. *Introduction to Psychology*, 7th Edn. Southbank, VIC: Thomson Wadsworth, 2005.

Poniewozik, James. "'West Wing': Terrorism 101", *Time*, Thursday 4 October 2001, available at http://www.time.com/time/printout/0,8816,178042,00.html, retrieved on 17 September 2009.

Prager, Jeffrey. "Healing from History: Psychoanalytic Considerations on Traumatic Pasts and Social Repair", *European Journal of Social Theory*, 2008, 11(3), 405-420.

Prince, Stephen. *Firestorm: American Film in the Age of Terrorism*. New York: Columbia University Press, 2009.

Proyas, Alex (director); O'Barr, James (comic book writer) and Schow, David J. (screenplay). *The Crow*. Santa Monica, CA: Crowvision Inc., 1994.

Puar, Jasbir. "On Torture: Abu Ghraib", *Radical History Review*, 2005, 93, 13-38.

Puar, Jasbir. *Terrorist Assemblages: Homonationalism in Queer Times*. Durham: Duke University Press, 2007.

Purvis, Neal and Wade, Robert (screenplay). *Casino Royale*. Los Angeles: Metro-Goldwyn-Mayer [MGM], 2008.

Rapoport, David. "Fear and Trembling: Terrorism in Three Religious Traditions", *American Political Science Review*, 1984, 78(3), 658-677.

Rapoport, David. "The Four Waves of Modern Terrorism", in Dipak K. Gupta, *Terrorism and Homeland Security*. Belmont: Thomson Wadsworth, 2006, 9-37.

Rauchway, E. "The President and the Assassin", *The Boston Globe*, 7

September 2003, available at http://www.boston.com/news/globe/ideas/articles/2003/09/07/the_president_and_the_assassin/, retrieved on 15 April 2005.

Rembrandts. "I'll Be There For You", theme music to *Friends*, lyrics available at http://www.lyricsondemand.com/onehitwonders/illbethereforyoulyrics.html, retrieved on 8 July 2008.

Reuter, Timothy. "Lessons of Terror: A History of Warfare Against Civilians: Why It Has Always Failed and Why It Will Fail Again – Recent Books", *SAIS Review*, Summer-Fall, 2002, 371.

Richardson, Louise. *What Terrorists Want: Understanding the Terrorist Threat.* London: John Murray, 2006.

Riessman, Catherine Kohler. *Narrative Analysis.* Newbury Park: Sage, 1993.

Rogers, Troy. "Seth McFarlane, American Dad Interview", *UGO.com*, http://www.ugo.com/ugo/html/article/?id=17297, no date, retrieve on 8 September 2009.

Rosen, Barry. "The Media Dilemma and Terrorism", in Yonah Alexander and Richard Latter (eds.), *Terrorism & the Media: Dilemmas for Government, Journalists & the Public.* Washington: Brassey's, 1990, 57-60.

Roth, Michael S. *Memory, Trauma and the Construction of History.* New York: Columbia University Press, 1995.

Rowe, Ryan; Solomon, Ed and August, John (writers). *Charlie's Angels.* Los Angeles: Columbia Pictures Corporation, 2000.

Roy, Arundhati. "L'Empire n'est pas invulnerable", *Manière de Voir*, 2004, 75(June-July), 63-66.

Rule, Audrey C. "An Analysis of Dollhouse Story Themes and Related Authentic Learning Activities", *Journal of Authentic Learning*, 2005, 2(1), 61-79.

Sardar, Ziauddin and Davies, Merryl Wyn. *Why Do People Hate America?* Duxford: Icon Books, 2002.

Sardar, Ziauddin and Davies, Merryl Wyn, *Will America Change?* Thriplow: Icon Books, 2008.

Savitch, H.V. "Does 9-11 Portend a New Paradigm for Cities?", *Urban Affairs Review*, 2003, 39(1), 103-127.

Schechter, Danny. *WMD: Weapons of Mass Deception.* Canoga Park, CA: Cinema Libre, 2004.

Schmid, Alex and Jongman, A.J. *Political Terrorism: A New Guide to Actors, Authors, Concepts, Data Bases, Theories and Literature.* North Holland: Oxford, 1988.

Schrobsdorff, Susanna. "Sexy or Sadistic?", *Newsweek*, 6 March 2007, available at http://www.msnbc.msn.com/id/17490782/site/newsweek/, retrieved on 8 May 2007.

Seib, Philip. *The Al Jazeera Effect: How the New Global Media are Reshaping World Politics.* Washington D.C.: Potomac, 2008.

Sengupta, Somini. "At Least 100 Dead in India Terror Attacks", *The New York Times*, 26 November 2008, available at http://www.nytimes.com/2008/11/27/world/asia/27mumbai.html, retrieved on 15 March 2010.

Sheer, Robert. *The Pornography of Power: Why Defense Spending Must be Cut.* New York: Twelve, 2008.

Sidibe, Gabourey, available at http://digg.com/celebrity/Precious_Star_Gabourey_Sidibe_The_Money_Shot_Dsheray_Dis?utm_source=feedburner&utm_medium=feed&utm_campaign=Feed%3A+digg%2Ftopic%2Fcelebrity%2Fupcoming+(Upcoming+in+Celebrity), retrieved on 9 March 2010.

Sienkiewicz, Matt and Marx, Nick. "Beyond a Cutout World: Ethnic Humor and Discursive Integration in *South Park*", *Journal of Film and Video*, 2009, 61(2), available at http://muse.jhu.edu/journals/journal_of_film_and_video/v061/61.2.sienkiewicz.html, retrieved on 23 March 2010.

Simmel, Georg. "The Metropolis and Mental Life", in *On Individuality and Social Forms: Selected Writings*. Chicago: The University of Chicago Press, [1903] 1971.

Singh, Baljit. "An Overview", in Yonah Alexander and Seymour Finger (eds.), *Terrorism: Interdisciplinary Perspectives*. New York: John Jay Press, 1977, 6-17.

Sixel, L. "EEOC Suit Claims Firing Prompted By Terrorism Fear", *Houston Chronicle.*, 2004, available at http://www.chron.com/cs/CDA/printstory.mpl/business/sixel/206095, retrieved 22 March 2004.

Sleeman, J. *Thugs; Or a Million Murders*. London: S. Low and Marston, 1933.

Smith, Nicola and Grimston, Jack. "European Police Probe Sex-Abuse Allegations in "Second Life"", *The Times*, 21 May 2007, available at http://www.foxnews.com/story/0,2933,273613,00.html?sPage=fnc.technology/videogaming, retrieved on 28 May 2007.

Solomon, Alisa. "Terror Attack", *The Village Voice*, 11 September 2001, available at http://www.villagevoice.com/2001-09-11/news/terror-attack/1, retrieved on 30 April 2010.

Sontag, Susan. "What Have We Done?" *The Guardian*, 23 May 2004, G2, 3-4.

Sorkin, Aaron (writer). "Isaac and Ishmael", *The West Wing*, season three, episode 0, clip available at http://www.youtube.com/watch?v=NDsY8qCxLHQ, retrieved on 4 September 2009.

Stallone, Sylvester and Lettich, Sheldon (writers). *Rambo III*. Culver City, CA: Tri Star Pictures, 1988.

Star, Darren (creator). *Sex and the City* [television series 1998-2004]. New York: HBO, 1998.

Stewart, John. "The Daily Show – First Broadcast After 9/11", available at http://www.buzznet.com/www/search/videos/speech/3401696/daily-show-first-broadcast-after/, retrieved on 4 September 2009.

Street and Smith's Sports Business Daily. "Nike Rolling Out New "Witness" Campaign Around LeBron James", available at http://www.sportsbusinessdaily.com/article/112472, retrieved on 22 February 2010.

Sumner, Tim. "Capt. Burke Died on 9/11 at the Hands of "Enemy Combatants"", *9/11 Families for a Safe & Strong America*, 2007, available at http://www.911familiesforamerica.org/?p=341, retrieved on 10 July 2008.

Swanson, David. "Is Best Antiwar Voice on TV Glenn Beck?" *American Chronicle*, 18 April 2010, available at http://www.americanchronicle.com/articles/view/151804, retrieved on 21 April 2010.

Sztrompka, Piotr. "Cultural Trauma: The Other Face of Social Change", *European Journal of Social Theory*, 2000, 3(4), 449-466.

Szymanek, Lukas. ""Friends" Not Forever in Television", *Lumino Magazine*, 15 April 2004, available at http://www.luminomagazine.com/mw/content/view/921/4, retrieved on 7 July 2008.

Taylor, Michael (writer) and Nankin, Michael (director). "The Ties That Bind", *Battlestar Galactica*, episode three, season four. Hollywood: Universal Studios, 2008.

Taylor, Paul A. "Pornographic Barbarism and the Self-Reflecting Sign", *International Journal of Baudrillard Studies*, 2007, 4(1), available at http://www.ubishops.ca/BaudrillardStudies/vol4_1/taylor.htm, retrieved on 31 January 2007.

Tester, Keith. "Bauman's Irony" in Anthony Elliott (ed). *The Contemporary Bauman*. London: Routledge, 2007, 81-98.

TISM. "Play Mistral For Me", *TISM*, from the album *Macchiavelli and the Four Seasons*. Northcote, VIC: Shock Records, 1995.

Toffoletti, Kim. *Cyborgs and Barbie Dolls: Feminism, Popular Culture and the Posthuman Body*. London: I.B. Tauris, 2007.

Toolis, Kevin. "Rise of the Terrorist Professors", *New Statesman*, 14 June 2004, available at http://www.newstatesman.com/print/200406140015, retrieved on 5 March 2010.

Tulloch, John. *One Day in July: Experiencing 7/7*. London: Little, Brown, 2006.

Tumarkin, Maria. *Traumascapes: The Power and Fate of Places Transformed by Tragedy*. Carlton, VIC: Melbourne University Press, 2005.

Turner, Bryan. *Vulnerability and Human Rights*. Pennsylvania: The Pennsylvania State University Press, 2006.

Turner, Chris. *Planet Simpson*. London: Ebury, 2005.

Turner, Graeme. "Tabloidisation, Journalism and the Possibility of Critique", *International Journal of Cultural Studies*, 1999, 2, 59-76.

Turner, Graeme. *Understanding Celebrity*. Los Angeles: Sage, 2004.

Turner, Graeme. "The Mass Production of Celebrity: "Celetoids", Reality TV and the "Demotic Turn"", *International Journal of Cultural Studies*, 2006, 9, 153-165.

TV.com. "The One Where Rachel Tells...", *TV.com*, 2008, available at http://www.tv.com/friends/the-one-where-rachel-tells.../episode/73775/summary.html, retrieved on 4 May 2008.

Urry, John. *Mobilities*. Cambridge, UK: Polity, 2007.

Versluys, Kristiaan. *Out of the Blue: September 11 and the Novel*. New York: Columbia University Press, 2009.

Virilio, Paul. *Ground Zero*. London: Verso, 2002.

Wachowski, Andy and Wachowski, Lana (directors). *The Matrix*. Hollywood, CA: Silver Pictures, 1999.

Wachowski, Andy and Wachowski, Lana (screenplay writers). *V For Vendetta*. Burbank: Warner Bros. Pictures, 2005.

Waitzkin, Howard and Magaña, H. "The Black Box in Somatization: Unexplained Physical Symptoms, Culture, and Narratives of Trauma", *Social Science and Medicine*, 1997, 45(6), 811-825.

Waugh, Jr., William. *International Terrorism: How Nations Respond to Terrorists*. Salisbury: Documentary Publications, 1982.

Waugh, Jr., William. *Terrorism and Emergency Management*. New York: Marcel Dekker Inc., 1990.

Weinberg, Leonard; Pedahzur, Ami and Hirsch-Hoefler, Sivan. "The Challenges of Conceptualizing Terrorism", *Terrorism and Political Violence*, 2004, 16(4), 777-794.

Weimann, Gabriel and Winn, Conrad. *The Theatre of Terrorism: Mass Media and International Terrorism*. New York: Longman, 1994.

Weinberger, Eliot. *9/12: New York After*. Chicago: Prickly Paradigm Press, 2003.

Weir, Peter (director). *The Truman Show*. Hollywood: Paramount Pictures, 1998.

West, Brad. "Collective Memory and Crisis: The 2002 Bali Bombings, National Heroic Archetypes and the Counter-narrative of Cosmopolitan Nationalism", *Journal of Sociology*, 2008, 44, 337-353.

West, Kelly. "TV Recap: Dollhouse: True Believer", 2009, available at http://www.filmhobbit.com/television/TV-Recap-Dollhouse-True-Believer-16144.html, retrieved on 22 February 2010.

West, Darrell and Orr, Marion. "Managing Citizen Fears: Public Attitudes Toward Urban Terrorism", *Urban Affairs Review*, 2005, 41(1), 93-105.

Whedon, Joss (creator and writer). "Ghost", *Dollhouse*, episode one, season one. Beverley Hills: Twentieth Century Fox, 2009.

Whedon, Joss (creator) and Minear, Tim (writer). "True Believer",

Dollhouse, episode five, season one. Beverley Hills: Twentieth Century Fox, 2009.

Whittaker, David. *Terrorism: Understanding the Global Threat*. Harlow, UK: Pearson Longman, 2007.

Whittington, Lewis. "Sex and the City – The Final Season", *Culturevulture. net: Choices for the Cognoscenti*, no date, available at http://www. culturevulture.net/Television/SexandtheCity.htm, retrieved on 8 July 2008.

Williams, Clive. *Terrorism Explained: The Facts About Terrorism and Terrorist Groups*. Sydney: New Holland, 2004.

Wolfe, Alan. "The Home Front: American Society Responds to the New War", in James F. Hoge, Jr. and Gideon Rose (eds.). *How Did This Happen?: Terrorism and the New War*. New York: Public Affairs, 2001, 283-294.

Zachurski, Emma. ""American Dad": An Unpromising Start for a Rehash Program", *Silver Chips Online*, 14 February 2005, available at http:// silverchips.mbhs.edu/story/print/4898, retrieved on 8 September 2009.

Ziffer, Daniel. "Australian TV Viewers Too Scared to Look Away", *The Age*, 21 July 2006, 7.

Zinn, Howard. *Terrorism and War*. Crows Nest, NSW: Allen & Unwin, 2002.

Žižek, Slavoj. "You May!", *London Review of Books*, 1999, 21(6), 3-6, available at http://www.lrb.co.uk/v21/n06/slavoj-zizek/you-may, retrieved 11 December 2007.

Žižek, Slavoj. *The Ticklish Subject: The Absent Centre of Political Ontology*. London: Verso, 1999.

Žižek, Slavoj. *Enjoy Your Symptom! Jacques Lacan in Hollywood and Out*, 2nd edn. New York: Routledge, 2001.

Žižek, Slavoj. *On Belief*. London: Routledge, 2001.

Žižek, Slavoj. *Welcome to the Desert of the Real!: Five Essays on September 11 and Related Dates*. London: Verso, 2002.

Žižek, Slavoj (ed). *Everything You Always Wanted to Know About Lacan (But Were Afraid to Ask Hitchcock)*. London: Verso, 2002.

Žižek, Slavoj. "The Matrix: Or, Two Sides of Perversion", in William Irwin (ed), *The Matrix and Philosophy: Welcome to the Desert of the Real*. Chicago: Open Court, 2002.

Žižek, Slavoj. *Organs Without Bodies: On Deleuze and Consequences*. New York: Routledge, 2004.

Žižek, Slavoj. *The Metastases of Enjoyment: Six Essays on Women and Causality*. London: Verso, [1994] 2005.

Žižek, Slavoj. *The Pervert's Guide to Cinema: Parts 1, 2, 3*. London: A Lone Star, Mischief Films, Amoeba Film Production, 2006.

Žižek, Slavoj. *The Parallax View*. Cambridge, MA: The MIT Press, 2006.

Žižek, Slavoj. *The Universal Exception: Selected Writings, Volume Two.* London: Continuum, 2006.

Žižek, Slavoj. "Foreword: Trotsky's *Terrorism and Communism*, or, Despair and Utopia in the Turbulent Year of 1920", in Leon Trotsky *Terrorism and Communism: A Reply to Karl Kautsky.* London: Verso, 2007, vii-xxxiv.

Žižek, Slavoj. *Violence: Six Sideways Reflections.* New York: Picador, 2008.

Žižek, Slavoj. *First As Tragedy, Then As Farce.* London: Verso, 2009.

Zurawik, David. "Era of Smiles Fading Away", *Baltimore Sun*, 2 May 2004, available at www.baltimoresun.com/entertainment/tv/bal-as.friends02may02,0,1061507.story, retrieved on 7 July 2008.

Index

Abu Ghraib 23, 29, 114-115, 183, 187-190
Afghanistan
    counterterrorism 132; democratic rights in 196; opium cultivation 129; in *Rambo III* 129; Russian invasion 129, 173; the spectacle of violence in 24; television audiences 95; terrorism in 65; war in 58, 115, 131, 141, 150, 197
Agamben, Georgio 127
Age, The 43, 45, 68, 181, 187
Alias 25, 168-169
allegory 26-27, 118, 158, 213-214, 222
al-Qaeda 71-72, 75, 129, 172, 217
American Dad 28, 32, 90, 151, 158-160, 164, 166
American Psycho (2000) 199
Angel 32
anxiety
    in the city 56, 101; and drama 95; fear and 23-24, 43, 52-53, 92, 148, 175; pornography and 176; terror and 20, 118, 145, 148; trauma and 96; and visual culture 74, 105
Australian, The 43, 69

Bali bombings 50, 81
banality
    celebrity 66; obscene 188;

routines 53, 58, 140, 182, 212; in screen cultures 29; sex and porn 184, 200; spectacles 183-186, 212; terrorism 62; the thing 153
Battlestar Galactica 5, 28, 32, 111-133, 211-212, 218
Baudrillard, Jean 17, 27, 35-38, 95-96, 154, 178-182, 188, 199-200, 212, 218
Bauman, Zygmunt 40, 91, 93, 99
Beck, Glenn 169
Beck, Ulrich 148
black museum of journalism 190
blogosphere 18, 27, 62, 64-65, 75-77, 136, 223
Buffy 32
Bully Beatdown 119
Bush, George W. 8, 21, 31, 71, 124, 171-172
business 55, 58, 123, 131
Butler, Judith 203-204

cat's cradle games 8
celebrity culture 4, 7, 27, 61-85
Chappelle, Dave 126
Chomsky, Noam 21, 29, 115, 128-129, 145, 210-211
Churchill, Ward 59, 98, 130, 140, 165, 224
cities
    fear and anxiety 23; Caprica 116; and images 31, 34, 36, 39; and the desert of the real

54-60; and the imagination 221; and newspapers 79; and power infrastructure 142; as terrorist training grounds 130; as a traumascape 40-42; and walls 131; and *we* 20, 23; and witnesses 54-60, 70, 208, 223

commodity 184, 190, 192, 198-200

Cordesman, Anthony 171

counterterrorism
conferences 118, 197; experts 218-219; and Hollywood 218; images of 185, 212; and Imaginationland 214-216; laws 167; and nudity 187; policing 79, 183; practitioners and academics 142; television 184, 218; and traditional research 32; and *24* 61, 65, 75, 83-84, 223; and witnesses 6

Crow, The (1994) 158

culture of terrorism
Chomsky 29, 115; screen culture 203-224

Debord, Guy 221

desert of the real 27, 33-60, 137

disavowal viii, 92, 97, 108, 118, 155

Dollhouse 29, 32, 183, 190-196

Doonesbury 162-163

dramatization 94, 117

Egypt 62-63, 170

Eisenstein, Zillah 41, 196-197

emergent 22, 159

everyday life 41, 55, 66, 92, 94, 98, 106, 115, 140, 153, 160, 219, 221

Family Guy 5, 28, 90, 151, 158-161, 163-164, 166, 218

fear
and the Hashashin 11-13; in the human fleet 117, 120-121, 131; of Muslims 21, 23, 50-51, 69, 81, 123-124, 164-165, 215; and the Sicarii 11-13; and the Thuggee 11, 13

fiction 6, 26, 38, 64-65, 90, 94, 106, 160, 183, 189

Friends 5, 28, 32, 41, 70, 77, 89-109, 137, 139, 151, 212-213, 218

Fromm, Erich 41, 91, 94-95, 140

fundamental attribution error 122

Global Terrorism Research Centre (GTReC) 171

Ground Zero 23, 38, 100, 139, 155, 198, 208

Grosz, Elizabeth 100-101

Haraway, Donna 7-9, 19, 48

Hashashin 11-13

Heidegger, Martin 153

Herald Sun 43, 69, 79

Hilton, Paris 66-67, 70

Hollywood 10, 27, 37, 64, 76, 95, 132, 180, 183, 185, 189, 216-218

How I Met Your Mother 70-71, 90, 139, 212, 218

hyperreality 36, 39, 150, 178-179, 182, 221

Imaginationland 4, 213-216, 220

In the Shadow of No Towers 198

Iran 164

Iraq
Abu Ghraib 23, 29, 114, 183, 187, 190; and the American flag 89; and counterterrorism 132; democratic rights in 196; *Doonesbury* 162; everyday life in 41; hegemony 131; the spectacle of violence 24; terrorism in 20, 51, 65, 72; war in 58, 115, 150, 197

Irish Republican Army (IRA) 46-
47, 144-145
irony
    and allegory 25; and Osama bin
    Laden 59; and post-9/11 comedy
    157-163, 170-173; and *South Park*
    166; and the superhero 169; and
    Žižek 141

Jameson, Jenna 4, 198-201
jouissance 119, 131, 176

Kristeva, Julia 135; 221
KRS-One 165-166

La Femme Nikita (1990) 185
Laqueur, Walter 6, 11, 64, 177
Letterman, David 5, 135, 137-143,
    148, 163, 172
London
7/7 attacks 6, 42, 50, 58, 62-63;
    Insurge 57; The London Central
    Mosque 157; as a targeted city
    30, 56, 119, 215
Los Angeles
in *Alias* 170; and *Friends* 101; post-
    9/11 103; in *24* 84

McFarlane, Seth 158-160, 164, 166,
    173
Madrid 42, 53, 56-58, 63, 119
Manhattan
    in *Battlestar Galactica* 127; and
    everyday life 140; in *Friends* 4,
    28, 91-93, 96-103, 106-109; in
    images 185; and John Stewart
    149; and Kabul 141; and the 9/11
    roll call 31; post-9/11 208; in *Sex
    and the City* 99; as a terrorist
    target 34, 223; in *The Day the
    Earth Stood Still* 139; and the
    thing 154; witnesses of 32

Matrix, The (1999) 27, 35-37
Melbourne
    Dr Anthony Cordesman 171-
    172; and multiculturalism 80-
    81; newspapers 68, 79-81, 181;
    research 8; skyline 8, 30, 56; as
    a terrorist target 42; view of 30;
    and *West Wing* 137; witnesses in
    20, 39, 42-43, 46-55, 58, 123, 182
Miller, Toby 17, 98, 106, 140, 143,
    171, 207-208
modest witness 19, 48
Monash University 30
money shot 29-30
Mumbai 61-62, 77-78, 83

Nacos, Brigitte 17, 67-68
New York City
    and Caprica 127; Fire
    Department 103; and New
    Yorkers vii-viii, 20, 41, 91, 93,
    98-99, 102-103, 106, 138, 204-205,
    212-213, 220, 224; skyline 89,
    91, 95, 100, 102, 154, 207; Twin
    Towers (World Trade Center)

Obama, Barack 89, 105, 171-172
objective violence 111-117, 126,
    131-133, 168
obscenity
Abu Ghraib 23, 114, 188;
    jouissance 119; 9/11 26, 39, 180;
    pornography 181-182, 184;
    power 154; response to 9/11 34,
    131, 212, 221; visual culture 189
Oklahoma City 68, 223
O'Reilly, Bill 129, 147, 173
Osama bin Laden 59, 67-69, 154

passage à l'acte 141
perverse
    Abu Ghraib 190; sexuality 115;

unreason 33-34; vision 9
pornography
    and terrorism 19, 28-29;
    terrorsex 175-201; and
    voyeurism 4;
Pretty Woman (1990) 185

Rapoport, David 12-13
Rather, Dan 141-143, 173
Richardson, Louise 14-15, 177, 183
Riverbend 41
routines 41, 53, 95, 140, 147-148,
    183, 212
Ruby Ridge 195

second life 108, 200
Second Life Liberation Army (SLLA)
    200
Seinfeld 139
sex
    at Abu Ghraib 29; and celebrity
    67; *and the City* 70, 90, 95,
    99, 102, 139, 218; cyber- 38,
    92; and democracy 197; and
    Dollhouse 191-196; and the
    internet 180; *In the Shadow of No
    Towers* 198; and Jenna Jameson
    201; and Manhattan 98; and
    pornography 176-178, 181-182,
    200; and second life 200; sells
    29, 69, 212; and surveillance
    187-188; and torture 188-190;
    and violence 23, 183-187;
sexual decoys 196-197
Shanksville, Pennsylvania 4, 37, 91
shock and awe 204
Sicarii 11-13
Simpsons, The 5, 28, 90, 108, 151-
    157, 159-160, 173, 218
simulations 179
situated knowledges 48
South Park 5, 158-159, 166, 213-216,
    218

Spiegelman, Art 198
sport
    celebrities 71, 76; and
    counterterrorism conferences
    197; and hazing 115; stadiums
    43
subjective violence 113-116, 126,
    130-133
Sydney 42, 79

Team America: World Police (2004)
    28, 151, 159, 166-167, 170,
terrorism as spectacle 24
terrorsex 28-29, 175-201
theater of terror 10-11, 15, 27, 32,
    40, 43, 57, 62, 176
The Day the Earth Stood Still (2008)
    138-139
Thuggee 11, 13
trauma
    and absences 28, 90; in cities
    56, 70-71, 95-97, 101, 123;
    and comedy 18, 28, 135-173,
    212; locations of 39; in the
    Matrix 35; overwhelming
    39-40; and pornography 176;
    psychoanalysis 92, 98-99, 108,
    130, 222; of terrorism 31, 209
traumascape 4, 39-40, 46, 56, 98,
    137
Tulloch, John 6
Turner, Bryan 40, 59, 158
Turner, Graeme 65-66, 76-77, 24 25,
    64-65, 83-85, 90, 168, 184, 223
Twin Towers
    and *Battlestar Galactica* 127; and
    Baudrillard 38; as celebrities 70;
    in images viii, 37, 70, 139, 207;
    and irony 157; and KRS-One
    165; in social research 49; as a
    symbol 34, 56, 58; on television
    5, 24, 89-91, 95, 98, 100-102,
    107; and *The Simpsons* 155; and

terrorsex 182, 185, 190, 198; as things 154-155; and Toby Miller 17; and Ward Churchill 59, 130

uncanny 10, 90, 177
unconscious viii, 7, 119-121

victims
  celebrities as 71; in cities 33, 46, 57-58; and comedy 136, 146; of terrorism 11-16, 203, 223-224; of terrorsex 188; of war 132
Vietnam War 16
vision
  embodied 9; and technology 10; witnessing 7, 29
Vogue: Italia 29, 183-190, 212

Waco 193, 195
Washington DC 4, 31, 34, 37, 40, 58, 60, 63, 91, 117-118, 129, 138-139, 148
we
  audiences of terror 10, 29, 63-64, 97-98, 113, 147, 180; and comedy 136-137, 165; and everyday life 41; fetishist disavowal 108; I and 19; and hyperreality 179; jouissance 119, 154, 180; KRS-One 165-166; sociology of 20-25,
48, 157, 172; and trauma 28; and the unconscious 93-94, 148, 219; undifferentiated 220-222; and the unforeseen 3; and violence 146; as witnesses viii, 30-31, 33-34, 37, 50-51, 53, 55, 57, 76, 80-82, 109, 176, 186, 190, 204-205
women 198
West Wing, The 5, 46, 90, 95, 135, 137, 144, 176
World Trade Center (2006) 25

X-Files, The 3, 132, 160, 196

Žižek, Slavoj
  Abu Ghraib 187; commodities 38; the desert of the real 27, 36; divine violence 119; the hero 169; *International Journal of Žižek Studies* x; irony 141; jouissance 119; and 9/11 15; paranoiac fantasies 92; passage à l'acte 141; passion for the real 64, 84; popular culture 217-218; and pornography 176, 180-182; as a social theorist 91; subjective and objective violence 111-115, 126, 130-131; the thing 154; trauma 96-98, 150, 222

CPSIA information can be obtained at www.ICGtesting.com
Printed in the USA
LVOW082332221212

312814LV00004B/75/P

9 780982 806135